"Mum! He's My Dad!"

A Mother Overcoming Abuse by Her Intimate Partner

Deirdre Fennessy

Cover photograph by Jacqueline Brooks
Edited by Ruth Fae | Fae Blood Publications
Cover design and Interior formatting by Captured by KC Designs
ISBN: 978-1-7644420-0-8 First edition

National Library of Australia Cataloguing-in-Publication Data: A copy of this publication has been deposited with the National Library of Australia and the relevant state library as required under Australian legal deposit legislation. National Library of Australia Cataloguing-in-Publication entry.

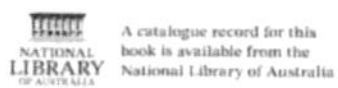
A catalogue record for this book is available from the National Library of Australia

Content Warning

This book has been written to raise awareness about hidden, unacknowledged trauma and how it can diminish our capacity to fully enjoy life. It also offers pathways toward healing and a sense of wholeness.

At times, there are detailed descriptions of intimate partner abuse, sexual assault, coercive control, childhood trauma, and systemic injustice. While these experiences are shared with positive intention, honesty, and care, please note they may be distressing or activating for some readers.

Please prioritise your wellbeing as you read. Take breaks, skip sections if needed, and seek support if anything in these pages feels overwhelming.

For a list of support services, please refer to the Resources section at the end of this book.

This is for all the abused women experiencing the effects of trauma from an intimate partner.

Contents

FOREWORD

by Moniquea Spiteri

WHEN I FIRST MET Deirdre, I was struck by her quiet determination. Beneath the grief and confusion that intimate partner abuse so often leaves in its wake, there was an unmistakable spark of courage, a readiness to face what had long been buried and to speak aloud what had once been unspeakable. As her therapist, I have had the privilege of walking beside her as she reclaimed her voice, her body, and her sense of belonging in the world.

What you hold in your hands is an act of reclamation. This book is both testimony and transformation that has been crafted through years of reflection, therapy, and embodied healing. It is the sound of a woman remembering her own truth after decades of silence.

Trauma, particularly the kind that unfolds within intimate relationships, is not only psychological, it is profoundly physiological. The body becomes the container for what the mind cannot yet face. It remembers everything: the moment the voice went quiet, the flinch, the freeze, the unbearable contradiction of loving someone who causes harm. The nervous system, in its infinite wisdom, protects us through patterns of numbness, appeasement, and disconnection. Healing, therefore, is not about forcing memories into words, it is about slowly creating safety in the body so that truth can emerge without retraumatisation.

Deirdre's work exemplifies this process. Through her willingness to tell her raw, unfiltered, and deeply human story, she offers her readers a bridge between silence and speech, between fragmentation and wholeness. As her writing evolved, I saw the unmistakable signs of integration: moments of tenderness amid rage, compassion where there had been self-blame, and an embodied sense of dignity where there had once been only trauma.

Telling one's story after trauma is tough. It requires immense courage to revisit what the body has tried to forget, and a deep well of self-compassion to stay present with one's own pain. It is also a profoundly political act, because every time a woman breaks her silence about coercive control, sexual violence, or psychological abuse, she challenges the systems that have normalised those harms. Each act of truth-telling begins to unravel the shame that binds generations.

As a somatic psychotherapist, I have spent many years supporting people through the slow, sacred work of trauma recovery. Healing is not the erasure of the past, it is the capacity to meet the past differently. It is when a victim's story no longer hijacks their nervous system but becomes part of an integrated narrative, when the body no longer tenses in anticipation of harm but begins to trust safety again. This transformation cannot be achieved through intellect alone, it arises through the body's gradual restoration of rhythm, breath, and connection. Deirdre's writing embodies this truth.

There is a visceral honesty in her words that reminds us trauma is not abstract because it lives in real bodies, families, and communities. Her story will resonate with anyone who has ever felt invisible, silenced, or blamed for their own pain. It also speaks to those who accompany those seeking to overcome trauma—the loved ones, clinicians, and advocates who must learn to listen without judgement and to hold space without rushing to fix.

What makes *"Mum, He's My Dad!"* so powerful is its layered truth. It is both deeply personal and profoundly universal. It exposes the hidden dynamics of coercion and control that can exist behind closed doors, even in relationships that appear "normal." It reveals the long shadow such trauma casts across the body and across generations, while also illuminating the possibility of repair. Deirdre writes not from bitterness but from a place of fierce compassion and integrity.

For readers who carry their own history of trauma, I offer this gentle reminder: Move through this book at your own pace. Notice your breath, your body, your heart. If the words ever feel too heavy, pause. Step outside, stretch, or place a hand on your chest and remind yourself that you are here, now, safe. Healing happens in small doses, in moments of truth met with equal moments of care. Let this story accompany you, not overwhelm you.

For those reading from a place of empathy or curiosity, I invite you to listen beyond the narrative and sense the resilience that pulses beneath each chapter. This is not a tale of victimhood. It is a chronicle of reclamation that reminds us that healing is possible, that the nervous system can find its way back to balance, and that even after profound violation, the human spirit can rise with dignity intact.

In a world where women are still too often silenced, disbelieved, or pathologised for naming abuse, Deirdre's voice joins a growing chorus that insists on truth. Her courage to write this book is a gift, not only to those who have endured similar pain but to the broader collective longing for justice and understanding.

May you approach these pages with compassion, for Deirdre, for yourself, and for the parts of humanity still learning what love truly means. Allow her story to touch you as a reminder of our shared fragility *and* our shared capacity to heal.

This book is a testament to what happens when silence is broken, when a woman's voice is reclaimed, and when the body can, at last, exhale.

Moniquea Spiteri

*Somatic Psychotherapist and certified Somatic Experiencing®
Practitioner Founder, Somatic Synergy and host of the Transcending Trauma® Podcast*

PREFACE

I Am Woman

BACK IN 1972, WHEN I was an innocent twelve-year-old, the classic number one hit single *I Am Woman,* sung by Helen Reddy and co-written by Reddy and Ray Burton, hit the airways. At that time, I was ignorant of the necessity for the message. Now, over fifty years later, its lyrics resolutely epitomise female solidarity and empowerment, and my conviction to make a huge noise calling for change about equality for women.

I am, however, saddened that when endeavouring to receive copyright permission from Universal Music Group in the USA, who own the rights to the lyrics, I was denied usage with no reason given. The late Helen Reddy, I imagine, would have wanted the message of her campaign to have been used for the continued effort for women's empowerment.

Nevertheless, we will get around this disappointment and utilise modern technology to access the lyrics. Please use the QR Code below to access Helen Reddy performing her classic hit single *I am Woman* and soak up the thought-provoking lyrics by referring to them throughout the book and at the end of each chapter.

In contrast was my desire to use the lyrics of *Edge Of Something*, co-written by Missy Higgins, Matteo Zingales, and Antony Partos. This is a contemporary song about women's empowerment—one that strengthens us against the setbacks and difficulties of life. I am immensely grateful that all three writers have kindly given me permission to use the lyrics of their hit song. Lyrics set to music are impactful to our emotions and can create change within us that other forms of media don't achieve. I'm indebted to be able to use the gift these artists have given us to help bring about change within our society. Thank you for allowing your creation to be part of this work.

Women in our society are flexing their vocal cords against the perceived notion that the female gender is inferior to our male brothers. Even though we serve humankind in a specific biological way in the reproduction of our species, we are not subordinate! Our reproductive role shouldn't mean that we are to be exploited, or expect to be seen as the second-rate gender; rather we should be valued and supported in our role as child nurturers. However, our role in advancing our species isn't restricted to just child nurturing, as our abilities, talents, and ideas complement those of our male counterparts. Despite some progress in the equality of gender, such as success in gaining the right to vote and working towards equal pay and job opportunities, many women throughout generations have been subservient to their male partners when it comes to sexual behaviour. Male sexual dominance has largely been kept secret from the wider community due to the supposition that it was a taboo subject and not for general discussion. In Australia, it has only been since the Royal Commission into Institutional Responses to Child Sexual Abuse (15 December, 2017), established by then Prime Minister, Julia Gillard, that much of the silence of victims (at least those still alive), has now been broken by utilising that platform. Now victims have been heard and believed. Their sad and, in most cases, life destroying experiences at the hands of perpetrators—often those in roles of trust—have been revealed. As a consequence of this trust being taken advantage of, devastating effects have been sustained on victims' mental health, relationships, and other life problems. Furthermore, the *#MeToo* movement brought to light the revelations of so many women exploited by work colleagues. Typically, these women were coerced or forced by blackmail into granting sexual favours to be able to advance their careers. Since 2006, this movement has revealed secrets of abuse of countless women from all walks of life. These ongoing revelations from both the Royal Commission and the *#MeToo* movement have continuously exploded through the media.

Due to my own experience of being controlled and manipulated by a sexually dominating male partner, which resulted in adverse effects to my mental health and my relationships with my children, I went looking for stories of other similar victims of Intimate-Partner Violence (IPV). I wanted to know how their lives were affected, more particularly if they were able to heal from the pain, and if so, how they managed their recovery. What surprised me was that while I found many examples of childhood abuse stories, I was dismayed to discover a total lack of stories about abuse of adult female victims at the hands of their perpetrator intimate male partners.

This made me wonder: *What is the real truth about women suffering in silence? What are the real numbers of vic-*

tims who are too embarrassed of their perceived shame to reveal their experiences? And are these victims getting help?

After struggling for many years with depression and anxiety, and ultimately being diagnosed with Post Traumatic Stress Disorder (PTSD), I knew I had to find a way to get back to wanting to live. Bottling it all in and trying to ignore the symptoms certainly wasn't working for me. I read what I could and utilised life experiences and professional help to work through strategies to make progress with recovery and healing. The more I read, the more I understood that keeping silent about abuse was not the means of achieving healing.

Speaking out and sharing my experiences was part of the answer to a wholesome, long-lasting recovery. I wanted to be part of the ever-increasing voice of women; to make a difference in that struggle for change. Recovery from abuse, especially sexual abuse and coercive control from a person you should have been able to trust, is incredibly difficult, particularly if you are caring for children at the same time.

As a collective cohort, women need to make noise. We need to be loud. We need to combine our resources of life experiences to encourage change in society, particularly in the behaviour of males. All of us should call out bad behaviour when we see and hear it. We need to share our successful strategies for recovery and healing from abuse so other women and their children can also succeed in their own recovery and healing. It is only by being vocal that society will be educated. This will bring greater awareness to the damage inflicted on women's lives, including the damage to their children.

In her acceptance speech when receiving the Australian of the Year Award for 2021, Australian activist and advocate Grace Tame said, "When we share, we heal... Every voice matters... Our voices are changing history... Let's make some noise, Australia!"

Sadly, the momentum has been slow since *I Am Woman* was first released in 1972, but with the courageous, determined voices of people like Grace Tame, awareness will continue to rise and change will happen.

I want to add my voice to the growing number making that noise. I want my sharing to help with attaining healing for traumatised women and for myself.

I want to be part of changing history that achieves making a difference for women to be treated better than I was. I want my voice to be loud for countless women who are too scared to "roar."

So, hear me roar!

...roar

...ignore

...pretend

...before

...floor

...again.

1

FUCK DIGNITY

"But now she was suddenly filled with a passionate desire to share everything, to say the bare ugly truth, to hold nothing back. Fuck dignity... This can happen to anyone."
—Liane Moriarty, *Big Little Lies*

VOICES OF WOMEN ARE now being heard loud and clear around the world, provoking a community shift in what is considered to be acceptable behaviour by men towards women. In 2017, American journalists Jodi Kantor and Megan Twohey broke the story about the coercive, manipulative, and controlling sexual abuse perpetrated by Hollywood producer Harvey Weinstein against actors and staff. The floodgates opened, and society's longstanding tolerance of men's unchallenged supremacy over women began to crumble. Then in 2006, Tarana Burke—a Black American woman from the Bronx, New York, who has advocated for over three decades for marginalised people, especially Black women and girls who have experienced sexual violence—started using the hashtag *#MeToo*.

Her intention was to enable women and girls to communicate in this way to gain empathy and support from each other while on their healing journey, and the movement quickly found global recognition. As more and more women used the hashtag to reveal their often long kept secrets, they brought into the daylight men's control over them to gain sexual favours by means of coercive manipulation or non-consensual intercourse, which—put simply—is rape. The silence was ruptured.

On Monday November 9, 2020, Australian *Four Corners* aired the episode "Inside the Canberra Bubble," reported by Louise Milligan, which highlighted investigations into the behaviour of some of our country's senior politicians. The high standard of integrity and proper conduct toward women that everyday Australians expect from their leaders was torn to shreds as stories of assault and abuse came to light. Eyewitness accounts disclosed partying politicians and staffers who, while living away from home, had too much alcohol and consequently behaved inappropriately in public.

The notion of "What happens in Canberra stays in Canberra" was challenged. If our country's "Capitol Hill" workplace was behaving inappropriately, what imperative was there for any workplace around our nation to comply with social expectations and moral standards?

Furthermore, in February of 2021, former Liberal Party staffer Brittany Higgins publicly alleged she had been raped in March 2019 by a colleague in the Parliament House building while being helped home after an alcohol-fuelled night out. Community opinion fuelled by incessant media speculation became divided, and Brittany had to endure her allegations being danced around and constantly rehashed after she went public with her story. Naturally, all the media was interested in was the sensationalism of the story rather than the welfare of either of the parties concerned, particularly the complainant.

The case finally went to trial in October 2022, where Brittany suffered days of continual harassment while being cross-examined on every aspect of her life. This included what ensued during the alleged rape, her actions immediately after it had occurred, and even her actions months and years later. In contrast, Bruce Lehrmann, the named alleged rapist, pleaded "not guilty" and, as was his right, did not enter the witness box. The basis of our legal system is that the prosecutor must prove the truth of the allegations "beyond reasonable doubt," meaning the accused doesn't have to give sworn evidence.

The accused's barrister can attempt to discredit the victim, her allegations, and her ongoing behaviour—so dragging the poor person through a horrendous mental experience—while the accused can sit back and watch his alleged victim continue to suffer in the witness box. In this case, the jury was unable to reach a unanimous verdict for a few days before the unthinkable happened: One of the jury members was found to possess extraneous material over that which was provided as evidence during the proceedings, so the trial was aborted.

Initially, a retrial was announced for the following February, but due to serious concerns regarding the significant effect this could have on the mental health of Brittany Higgins, the prosecutor announced the abandonment of the case. This whole saga has highlighted the unfair bias in our legal system that effectively puts the onus on the complainant and the prosecutor to prove the guilt of the alleged perpetrator. As a result, victims are left vulnerable to aggressive cross-examination by the defendant's legal team, often with blatant disregard for the ongoing trauma this inflicts.

With so many victims unable to cope with ongoing trauma, many do not report their experience to police—and those who do report rarely get to a trial that results in a guilty verdict. Our legal system needs a complete overhaul to achieve better, more realistic outcomes that protect women from further trauma and result in justice and accountability. Even though a guilty verdict was never achieved in Brittany's case, this does not mean that something traumatic did not happen to her. Nevertheless, Brittany's bravery in going public exposed the misconduct of men in the highest workplace in our nation. Change will come only when men realise that they risk their conduct being exposed and that their careers may be destroyed by their actions.

The Australian of the Year (2021) was awarded to Tasmanian Grace Tame for her outspoken advocacy for victims of sexual assault to be permitted to speak publicly about their experience and their abuser, especially those victims abused in institutional locations. Groomed by her fifty-eight-year-old maths teacher at the age of fifteen, Grace had to endure her abuser bragging on Facebook about how awesome his exploits were after serving only nineteen months of his two-year, ten-month sentence. This gained him only another extra four months in jail! He enjoyed being interviewed by commentator and sex therapist, Bettina Arndt, where he portrayed himself as the victim by highlighting what he had lost in his life. But there was never any mention of an apology or acknowledgement of the damage he had caused to his victim. Grace decided it was time for her to hit back, break her silence, and speak about the effect and damage on her life from the abuse and the injustice of allowing him to speak about her story, all the while gloating about his exploits. An archaic law in Tasmania, however, prevented her from this course of action as it "gagged" her from being able to speak about her perpetrator and tell her story. A story, she said, that was "her story, one that she owned;" a narrative that she was being prevented from telling. Grace wanted to take back the control, so she started to campaign, using the slogan *#LetHerSpeak*.

It took her two years, but the Tasmanian Parliament finally changed the law, granting Grace the right to reveal her identity and break the silence. Her advocacy for victims earned Grace the Australian of the Year Award for 2021. In her acceptance speech she stated, "Trauma does not discriminate, nor does it end when the abuse itself does. Every voice matters. Just as the impacts of evil are borne by all of us, so too are solutions born of all of us."

By using her new platform, she has certainly kindled an on-going conversation that is stimulating change in society. Grace has continued her quest to keep communication on-going to breed better understanding in the belief that, as society gains the appreciation of victims' stories, more victims will be encouraged to end their silence. By sharing their stories, victims will ultimately achieve better healing and recovery for themselves and other victims. This will lay the foundation for progress in preventing further abuse with social reform.

Another advocate for societal and legal reform is Saxon Mullins, the Director of Advocacy at *Rape and Sexual Assault Research and Advocacy*. Appearing in 2018 on the *Four Corners* episode, "I Am That Girl," she revealed her identity along with her story about being raped in 2013 by Luke Lazarus in an alley behind his father's Kings Cross nightclub. Initially being found guilty of rape by a jury at his first trial, Lazarus was later found not guilty when the NSW Court of Criminal Appeal quashed the first verdict and ordered a retrial. This second trial resulted in a not guilty verdict on the grounds that Lazarus' belief that Mullins had consented constituted "reasonable grounds," and thus did not meet the legal definition of rape. The controversial retrial initiated a new conversation as to what is considered/meant by "sexual consent." In turn, this triggered a review of the NSW laws. Mullins' quest has been to advocate that a "freeze response" should not be construed as giving consent. She refused to remain silent as she is passionate about making a difference not only by reforming consent laws, but also societal views of what true consent means, to better protect and empower women and to educate young women and men alike.

When a woman who has a disability is dependent on a caregiver or family members for support, abuse seems even more difficult to fathom. When a partner exploits their position of power for personal gratification, they break the promise made in their marriage vows or commitment to love and treasure the other person. After experiencing physical, emotional, financial, and sexual abuse for over a decade, Nicole Lee first disclosed her plight to a nurse after trying to end her life and being admitted to hospital. Perceiving the reason behind her attempted suicide, the nurse asked if Nicole would like to go to a women's refuge. Other women in her situation would normally accept the offer, but Nicole, who used a wheelchair, was dependent on assistance for daily living that also included caring for her two young children. Not long after her disclosure, the nurse called her husband, who was her full-time carer, to come and collect her and take her home. Nicole stated:

> "That broke me down as a person, to be sent home to the house I was being abused in with the person I was being abused by. It was this sense of 'no one's going to be able to get me out, I've got no way of getting out of this.'"

She was "terrified" when, some time later, the police did remove her husband from the house. This safeguarded her from the abuse, but it left her with no carer to assist her to do the basic daily tasks for herself and her children. No one asked her what she needed. Her husband did plead guilty to the abuse and was sentenced to two and a half years in jail.

The Victims Survivors' Advisory Council—established by the Victorian Government and chaired by former Australian of the Year, Rosie Batty, following the recommendations that were handed down by the *Royal Commission into Family Violence*—has benefitted significantly from Nicole's appointment as one of the twelve members who have lived experience of family violence. Using her advocacy platform, Nicole speaks out against family violence by lobbying for change and assisting those experiencing family violence and abuse.

Gymnastics had been the pinnacle of author and journalist Lucia Osborne-Crowley's ambitions until, at fifteen, she was brutally raped by a total stranger while enjoying a relaxing night-out with friends. This culminated in crippling physical and psychological health issues for the next ten years that not only destroyed her gymnastics aspirations but nearly ended her life. It wasn't until she broke her silence of the memories that she had tried to erase for ten years, by blurting out the details of her harrowing encounter to a clinician, that the traumatic event was linked to her debilitating health problems. Sympathetic medical practitioners slowly started repairing the damage that ravaged her body and the cyclical, ongoing psychological impact of the trauma.

Documenting her story in her book, *I Choose Elena,* Osborne-Crowley succeeds in portraying the damage done to herself by not being aware of what trauma does to the body, and sets out her research into understanding the mission for recovery. She states in her conclusion:

I'm a writer. I can't change the world. What I can change is the size of silence. The weight of it. The way it pulls us under. Trying to erase this experience was the surest way to let it define me. I wish I had known that. But I didn't, and so I said nothing.

When I did find a way to tell the truth, it was too late. My intervention was impotent against a body frozen with fear and decayed by disease. Full recovery will never be possible for me because no one, least of all me, wanted to struggle with the listening or the telling. Because no one, least of all me, wanted to face the possibility that it was real. Because of my silence, the damage done to me is irreversible.

The truth of my life was expressed best by Chelsea Williams during the trial of Larry Nasser: *There will never be a time when I am not recovering. (Osborne-Crowley 2020, 137-38)*

These women have required heroic bravery to bare their stories in public, and I thank them immensely for doing so. By taking this action they have challenged the misguided perception of victims that silence and burying their pain was the only way to deal with abuse, and that one should just learn to bear the consequences of a troubled life.

Abuse can happen to anyone, anywhere; it happened to me when I least expected it and was perpetrated by the person I least expected it from. Just because I married the man I loved, he believed he had the marital right to get what he wanted, and he just took it. I carried my secret burden for decades before I sought any help.

Then when I did reveal my secret, I was humiliated and insulted with comments like: "You were married to him, you would have expected to have sex!" "That's life, you sometimes just have to suck it up!" and, "Why did you stay for so long if he was hurting you?"

Patricia A. Levesh, an attorney for the Greater Boston Legal Services sent a "Letter to the Editor" to the Boston Globe reflecting her thoughts on a common belief held in the community about victims of domestic abuse.

In part, her letter stated:

> Too often the victim is expected to leave the situation, so victims of domestic violence are essentially blamed for staying. We should never be asking why victims stay. The real question is why, as a society, do we continue to portray intimate victim violence as anything other than it is: a crime?

If the parties to an assault were not in a relationship, no one would ever suggest that the victim was to blame for permitting the assault to occur.

My experience working with victims of domestic abuse has shown me that society treats these crimes differently. Why else would the media persistently refer to an assault on one's partner as a "domestic dispute?"

It's a crime, and it needs to be treated as such. To do less is to perpetuate prejudice against victims, permit perpetrators to continue to deny responsibility, and allow the judiciary to impose sentences that send a message to perpetrators that it is not really a crime to beat up [or sexually abuse] your spouse.[1]

Society has buried its collective head in the sand and ignored this community travesty as being a problem that should stay private, behind closed doors.

What about all the poor women who have been murdered by their supposed trusted partners?

---

1. Levesh, Patricia A., "Letter to the Editor', Boston Globe, sec A, p 8. Published in 'No Place for Abuse, Biblical & Practical Resources to Counteract Domestic Violence', Kroeger, Catherine Clark & Nason-Clark, Nancy. *Words in [...] my addition.*

What about the child, or children, who are killed along with their mother, or left without a mother to nurture them and only a murderer for a father who should be in jail for life?

Either situation is a travesty beyond words!

The *Australian and Domestic and Family Violence Death Review Network Data Report: Intimate Partner Violence Homicides 2010-2018*, documents harrowing statistics. These statistics show that:

- 1 in 5 women and 1 in 20 men have endured some form of sexual abuse.

- Intimate partner homicide accounted for 21 percent of all homicides during the period of 2018-19.

- On average, 1 woman a week and 1 man a month are murdered by a current or a former intimate partner.

- The majority of the women killed experienced domestic violence from their intimate partner.

- When the offender was a woman, in the majority of the cases they were a domestic violence victim.

- Family and domestic violence deaths rarely occur without a period of an escalating pattern of behaviour of violence and coercive control.

- And when a woman does leave an abusive situation, this can be a more dangerous period for her safety.

Australia's National Research Organisation for Women's Safety (ANROWS), who reduce violence against women and their children, have used this Network Data Report to try and improve the work in protecting women and their children. A lot more work does need to happen.

Many of us who are lucky enough to be able to tell our stories use the word "survivor" to describe themselves. I hate using that word! In fact, I cringe every time I hear it used in the context of a victim of abuse being a "survivor." To me, it evokes the connotation that being a victim of sexual abuse has only two alternatives: that I will die due to being murdered by my abuser, or I will die by committing suicide, whichever happens first. Neither of which is the outcome any society would want for victims. "Survivor" should only apply when a person could have died after an event or incident. Keep the word for someone who nearly died from a plane or car crash, or a severe illness, or an operation.

A second meaning of the word "survivor" can be used to describe a person who has coped well and is unaffected despite a stressful period or difficulties in their life. Again, I feel this does not apply to sexual abuse victims. I don't think any victim who has had to put up with repeated abuse would have coped well and come through unscathed; or if they have been unaffected, then the abuse hasn't impacted their life to warrant the classification as a victim. I am not a survivor—I am a victim who has "endured" abuse and I'm "overcoming" or "conquering" that abuse. Call me a "sexual abuse overcomer" or a "sexual abuse conqueror."

In the same way as Osborne-Crowley declares, "I will always be recovering, it will always be ongoing," I am successfully overcoming and taking back control of my life, but the challenge and struggle is always going to continue; it will never go away. As Grace Tame said, the "trauma… doesn't end when the abuse does."

In her book *Big Little Lies*, Liane Moriarty doesn't hold back from portraying domestic violence and sexual abuse in society and its ramifications on women's lives. Two women in the story are abused. One is violently raped by a stranger who had started out being gentle and loving in a one-night-stand encounter that resulted in the conception of a child who never knew his father. The other is abused by her husband, who oscillates between being incredibly passionate and considerate and then the total opposite—extremely physically violent.

At the end of the novel, it is this latter character, the woman abused by her husband, who is about to speak at a forum of health professionals. The reason for the forum was for the audience to hear lived experiences of abuse, and so learn when to ask more questions of clients and to not ignore possible important signs of issues. She was planning to only tell them the bare facts of her domestic violence story without baring her soul. Her thoughts were, "She would keep her dignity. She would keep a little piece of herself safe. But now she was suddenly filled with a passionate desire to share everything, to say the bare ugly truth, to hold nothing back. *Fuck dignity!*" (*Moriarty 2018, 469*)

As she looks out over the audience, she spots a man looking terrified, obviously coming to terms with his own story of being the perpetrator and being asked to share. Suddenly, she wants him to know that she understood, "...all the perfect little lies he'd told himself for all those years, because she'd told herself the same lies. She wanted to enfold his trembling hands between her own and say, 'I understand'."

Then she finally began her speech by saying: *"This can happen—to anyone."*

I have been empowered by the courage of these women to break my silence and use my words and voice to share my experience of sexual abuse, and to be healed from the lies I had been telling myself about myself. I want the sharing of my trek to bring more awareness to the plight of abused women and break the culture of silence.

I want the children born by women who have been sexually abused by their husbands or intimate partners to explore their role, if any, to play a part in bringing about accountability and justice for their mothers.

I want the strategies that I found to be mightily successful in my evolution of healing to be utilised by others to transform their lives as well. I want a radical raising of the bar for women to obtain justice for the crimes committed against them (from the current miserable one percent conviction rate).

I want societal reform in the language used when speaking to or about victims. I want perpetrators to seek guidance to grasp the enormity of their faults. I want perpetrators to be accountable by first realising, and then admitting to, their abusive behaviour; for them to realise the damage they have caused, to give an apology, to seek forgiveness, and to change their ongoing behaviour.

I want perpetrators to change their conduct towards their victims in a way that will make victims feel respected and dignified. I want perpetrators to be part of the healing process for victims and for their own healing from their own guilt or perverted values. I want perpetrators to aid and encourage other perpetrators to be enlightened to reform.

I want my story, my trek, to open up dialogue that makes an impact for discussion and societal change.

So, just like Liane Moriarty's character in her book, I too want to share the bare ugly truth of my experience. Thus, I also say, "Fuck dignity."

...wise

...pain

... price

...gained

...anything.

2

#MeToo

"What I know for sure is that speaking your truth is the most powerful tool we all have."
—Oprah Winfrey at the Golden Globe Awards in 2018.

IT IS THE DREAM of most women to have children, and especially for some, to have a daughter. I was no different. My first child, my son Nathan, was a gorgeous fair-haired boy, nicknamed by my father as the "Duracell Kid" due to the fact that he never slowed down; a trait and gift he still has in his adult life. Then, sixteen months later, after a long, tough labour I was blessed with delivering a beautiful little girl—albeit with a "cone head" from the pressure of such a hard labour.

She was born in the evening and the following morning, after a much-needed sleep, the nurse brought Merryn in for me to feed her. I didn't have much trouble getting her onto the breast and my bonding with her was immediate. I thought she was absolutely beautiful, although she actually looked very strange with her narrow cone head contrasted by her chubby cheeks. But mothers can be blind when it comes to their baby and she was my longed for, much desired and beloved baby girl. As she contentedly slept in her cot, I gazed at her and marvelled at the miracle of the life I had birthed. I remember praying that I hoped that we would be great friends when she grew up, and that one day as a grandmother I would share the enjoyment of her children, too. I felt I could not be happier and more proud than I was at that moment.

Less than three years later my children-count doubled with my near-death experience of giving birth to adorable twin boys, Jared and Rohan. It took me nearly three weeks in hospital to recover enough to go home and start the mammoth task of looking after four pre-schoolers. My four children have been my life and focus—in doing all the things we do as mothers, I tried to put their welfare first in every decision and choice. It was paramount for me that they felt loved and nurtured, were safe, well educated, given many well-balanced life experiences, brought up in the Christian faith, had good morals taught and shown to them, and had good friends and extended family relationships. All this so they would grow up and live their adult lives making good choices for themselves and their families, and ultimately, give me much desired grandchildren to continue the miraculous cycle of life.

Nathan was the first to marry, followed about a year later by Merryn and, another year after that, by Rohan. A few years after that, Jared also married and I'm extremely fortunate to have one marvellous son-in-law and three delightful daughters-in-law.

Merryn was the first to give me a granddaughter, with two more granddaughters following nineteen and then twenty months apart. Privileged to be at the birth of the first and third babies, (I missed the second one because she arrived too quickly), it was incredible to witness my own grandchildren enter the world. Admittedly though, it was very stressful for me to see my own daughter in so much pain and discomfort. The first day Merryn was home with her firstborn, I received an SOS text early in the morning asking me to buy some cloth nappies as the baby was overflowing with milk and they had run out of mopping up cloths.

Over the next few years, there were numerous SOS calls, which I willingly and lovingly obliged. Spending a full day at their house doing the family washing, shopping, cooking meals, cleaning, and whatever else needed to be done was my pleasure, as this meant Merryn could be less stressed and more relaxed to enjoy her babies.

When my children were young I didn't have any family around me, as our families lived over a two hour drive away, so I had to do it all myself and rely on church friends to help when I was sick or needed to go to medical appointments. Knowing from experience just how stressful it is trying to keep up with all the demands of a young family, I wanted to alleviate as much of that stress from Merryn as I could. By contributing my time and effort, and babysitting often, I endeavoured to enable Merryn and her husband to spend some important alone-time together.

Merryn is a paediatric nurse, and she wanted to return to work for two shifts a fortnight once the babies were old enough to be left for the ten hours or so needed for a shift. So, Grandma stepped in to babysit. This also gave me time to bond with each of the girls and have them at my place and in my environment. I would read the various books and play the assorted games I had kept from when my children were small, just for this very time. My great enjoyment was to say to them, "Your mum used to play with this," or, "This was one of your uncle's favourite books." It was a special and precious time that I continue to treasure.

When Merryn was pregnant with her third child, she began to take the first two to *The Art Place*, a pre-school art and activity group held at the school the girls were going to attend (the same school that my children went to when we returned to Melbourne). Merryn asked if I could help her with the girls, and this became a special time with my daughter, the girls, and other mums and grandparents. It was stimulating to be creative, and many times I would feel excited that I was enjoying my third childhood. After the morning activities, I would usually help Merryn with tasks at her home. This continued for five years until her youngest started school.

As the girls grew older, I missed the time I spent with them as pre-schoolers. I continued to oblige, however, when Merryn called upon me to help with school or kindergarten pickup, or swimming lessons, or with after-school care until Merryn's husband got home from work. But then the school holidays became a time when all three children would need to be looked after for the whole day while both their parents were at work. Initially I thought I would cherish this time, but I found myself more and more unable to tolerate entertaining them and keeping the three of them occupied and away from upsetting each other. The more I was asked to look after all three of them together, the more I became stressed and anxious, and longed for the end of the day when they would go home. I wondered what was wrong with me. I had what I had longed for—to be a mother and a grandmother—but was struggling to enjoy it.

Merryn told me I was too strict with the girls and that I should slacken off my boundaries and relax more. She said to let them make a mess and have fun; not to be so obsessed with getting things done around the house, but just to enjoy spending time with them. To cope with the stress was all I wanted to do, yet I was finding that I was becoming overwhelmed, hating myself, and feeling extremely depressed and anxious.

Then, on the 5th October, 2017, the dam-wall broke with the story of Harvey Weinstein's perpetration of sexual harassment and abuse. Millions of women around the world started telling their stories of mistreatment and abuse. The *#MeToo* movement exploded, with women coming out of the woodwork to share long-buried trauma and haunting descriptions of their experiences. As more and more revelations came out with graphic details of the pitiful things men had done to women over so many years, I would just sit in front of the TV and cry and cry.

As my husband (my second marriage—not the father of my children) and I watched the revelations continually unfold I said to him, "If those women are suffering so much from a few episodes of sexual assaults, I must have so much suppressed trauma from being violently raped by my first husband on my wedding night, being raped repeatedly in my sleep, and the many attempted rapes and sexual assaults over the nearly eighteen years we were married."

Even though he was aware that I had been sexually abused during my first marriage, he was extremely shocked at my disclosure of the extent of the abuse, and the now-apparent effect being manifested in front of the TV. He insisted I go to the doctor to get a diagnosis of what appeared to be trauma symptoms, which I refused to do for quite a while as I didn't want to have to dig it all up again and deal with it. I felt I had successfully pushed it down, so it wouldn't need to be dealt with anymore. But my reactions grew progressively worse as the news continued to be full of more and more women and their heartbreaking stories about more and more men who, of course, denied, denied, denied.

The Royal Commission was also featured in the media at the time with horrific stories of mentally and emotionally damaged children, (now adults), and many accounts of other people ending their lives due to the shame and effect of the exploits of men who were supposed to be protecting them. This was a new world of exposure in which men were being challenged to give account for their actions and behaviour—and for people, especially women, to be able to tell their harrowing stories, be believed, and finally get some action.

Eventually, I did go to my doctor, who immediately diagnosed me with Post Traumatic Stress Disorder (PTSD) upon hearing only a small part of my story. She then helped me to make an appointment to see a counsellor at Eastern Centre

Against Sexual Assault (ECASA). After an initial appointment, possible avenues for recovery were discussed, one being to make a statement to the police and also to have continued counselling appointments (which I pursued for many years).

When Oprah Winfrey accepted the Cecil B. DeMille Award for lifetime achievement at the Golden Globes in 2018, just as the *#MeToo* movement was gaining its global momentum and influence, she delivered a powerful, gut-wrenching speech that produced a standing ovation:

> We also know it's the insatiable dedication for uncovering the absolute truth that keeps us from turning a blind eye to corruption and to injustice. To tyrants and victims and secrets and lies. I want to say that I value the press more than ever before as we try to navigate these complicated times, which brings me to this: What I know for sure is that speaking your truth is the most powerful tool we all have. And I'm especially proud and inspired by all the women who have felt strong enough and empowered enough to speak up and share their personal stories.
>
> Each of us in this room are celebrated because of the stories that we tell, and this year, we became the story. But it's not just a story affecting the entertainment industry. It's one that transcends any culture, geography, race, religion, politics, or workplace.

So, I want tonight to express gratitude to all the women who have endured years of abuse and assault because they, like my mother, had children to feed and bills to pay and dreams to pursue. They're the women whose names we'll never know.

I am one of those women and I have a name. I am now strong enough and empowered enough to speak up. I have a voice for women, for the truth to be told, to be heard and believed, to have my story, my "trek" told, and my case documented as a statistic. I desire justice and accountability to happen for abused women, especially those who have suffered Intimate Partner Violence (IPV) for crimes committed against them.

Subsequently, I did decide to make a statement to the police. This was a harrowing experience. Although it was one I felt I had no option but to do, considering my continuing PTSD and lack of any resolution to the historical and ongoing emotional abuse inflicted upon me by my ex-husband. It took the police over nine months to be ready to arrest my ex-husband and question him. Once he was contacted by the police, I knew my children, especially my daughter, would know (via their stepmother), and I knew that my life would be very different. But it was a risk I had no option to take if I was to have any chance of getting better.

Thus there was no surprise when I received that phone call from my daughter: "Mum! What do you think you are doing? What about forgiveness? What good will come of going to the police? He's my Dad!"

...strong
...invincible
...woman

3

TO LOVE AND TO CHERISH???

"...to have and to hold from this day forward, for better, for worse, for richer, for poorer, in sickness and in health, to love and to cherish, until we are parted by death. This is my solemn vow."
—Traditional wedding vow.

BRIAN AND I MET at a Uniting Church in Melbourne, where my sister and I grew up. Deciding it was time for him to make his own way, Brian had moved to the area when his father retired as a Uniting Church minister. Ours was a short courtship. I saw Brian as a quiet, gentle man who was set up well with a good career in instrumental engineering, and he had already secured a home loan with his own house. The most important part, though, was that I fell in love with him. The son of a clergyman! How lucky was I? So, when he proposed, I did not hesitate to say "Yes."

Brian had two married siblings—one who had been married for thirteen years and another who married earlier that year—as well as a younger brother who was engaged to be married later that year. As he was approaching his thirtieth birthday, he was keen to not feel left behind. So we set the date and started planning.

A couple from the *Navigators*, the Christian group Brian had been part of for about ten years, invited us to do a marriage preparation course with them. This was very helpful to understand the new relationship and adjustments that we would be encountering as a newly married couple. Our sexual relationship was a big part of this study. I wanted to keep my virginity for marriage and Brian respected that, but on occasion we did engage in petting as he was very keen to explore our sexuality. We had talked about sex and our desire for a healthy sexual relationship, and we were both keen for children.

We were married by his father and our local minister at noon on 31st October 1981 in a joyous celebration with many family and friends. Our lunchtime reception was held in the church hall, and finished in the late afternoon whereupon we left for the airport to commence our honeymoon in Tasmania. We shared joyously about how wonderful the day had turned out, fulfilling our dreams for the wedding we had wanted to celebrate our union.

Unfortunately our flight was delayed, and we experienced various other difficulties with finding our luggage and organising the hire car. So what we thought was a sensible move to start our honeymoon by flying to Launceston, ended up with us not arriving at our motel room until after eleven o'clock at night. Emotionally and physically exhausted, I communicated to Brian that I just wanted a shower and to fall asleep. Being a virgin, I wasn't in the best shape to embark on my first penetrative sexual experience. Although he made no verbal comment back to me, I believed that Brian was in agreement, but he obviously had other plans to deliberately ignore my wishes.

Exhausted, but feeling content from the most amazingly happy day, I was thankful to be finally lying in bed and I closed my eyes ready to go to sleep. Next thing I knew, I was suddenly uncovered, rolled on to my back, and my night gown was pulled up. I don't think he even removed my underwear but pulled it to the side. Brian's words were, "I know this is going to hurt you, but I just have to do it."

Without any foreplay or added lubricant he pinned my arms down and proceeded to forcefully insert his penis into my vagina. Begging him to stop as I tried to free myself from his grip, I remember looking over to the door of the motel room expecting someone to come in response to my screams.

But no-one did! The pain was immense; it felt like I was being ripped apart. It must have been only a minute or so before he ejaculated and flopped down on his side of the bed, stating, "I've waited a long time for that." Then he promptly rolled over away from me and, I presume, went to sleep. He didn't inquire how I was or check on my condition. He just rolled away and went to sleep.

The man who had promised to love and cherish me for the rest of our lives—a promise that was witnessed by our families and friends—categorically broke his promise that very same day, only a few hours after he had made it. In shock I just lay there, paralysed, until exhaustion took over and I fell asleep.

In the morning, Brian got up as if nothing had happened, and I was too scared to bring it up. We went down for breakfast and got on with the day. The rest of the honeymoon was spent travelling around Tasmania with Brian insisting on sex almost every morning and night. My body was extremely sore. Being too scared to refuse him, I could barely communicate with him and became very depressed.

In Hobart I remember trying to talk with him about my feelings, but it was as if he was closed to any idea that what he was doing was wrong. He just kept repeating, "Married couples have sex, that is what you do when you are married."

By the end of the honeymoon, he was refusing to even talk to me due to my despondent demeanour. The silent treatment had started. I was in shock, totally bewildered and confused about how to handle what I was experiencing. My expectations had been to have a caring husband who was going to love and cherish me for the rest of my life, but he had morphed into someone else and was no longer the man I had fallen in love with.

Looking back on this scenario, I am amazed and appalled that in 1981 in Victoria and Tasmania, it was not a crime to rape your wife. It only became subject to the Crimes Act as rape in Victoria in 1982 and in Tasmania in 1987.

A few days after our return from Tasmania, Brian had to travel overseas for work for three weeks. I basically reasoned away his behaviour, putting his thoughtless actions down to the fact he had to go abroad straight after the honeymoon. While he was gone and I was living in his house—living by myself for the very first time and feeling strangely alone—I promised myself that I would fulfil *my* marriage vow of, "For better or worse... until we are parted by death. This is my solemn vow." I felt I was damaged goods, and that if I didn't stay with him I may never have children. So, at the naïve age of twenty-one, I made a vow to myself to uphold the promise I had made to Brian only a few weeks before in the sight of God and in the presence of family and friends who witnessed those words on our wedding day. I decided I would do whatever it took to make this marriage work and bury the memory to keep my devastating experience a hidden secret.

So, on Brian's return from overseas I became his chattel, too scared to refuse his advances and simply hopeful for peace between us. Brian's work required him to do a lot of interstate travel and lengthy overseas trips, which wasn't a good fit for a married man, so he applied for a job with the Victorian State Electricity Commission (SEC). His application was successful, enabling us to have more stability.

I was desperate to start a family and thought that having children would bring us closer together. Brian was keen as well (I feel this was probably more to prove his manhood than anything else), and we were successful in falling pregnant just four months into the marriage. Nathan was born in December of 1982. I loved being a mother more than words can say. I would just gaze at the perfection that lay in my arms, suckled at my breast, slept soundly in his bassinet, or looked around taking in the world as I walked him in his pram.

The SEC asked Brian if he was prepared to do a secondment to the Latrobe Valley for three months, to work on the commissioning of the new coal-fired power station Loy Yang A. So when Nathan was four months old, we made what we thought would be a temporary move to Morwell in the Latrobe Valley, about two to three hours away from home and family.

Then, a few months into the secondment, an opportunity to remain there arose when the SEC was giving grants to engineers to encourage them to permanently move and work in the Latrobe Valley on the Loy Yang B project. Brian thought this would be a good opportunity for his career, and for us to bring our children up in a country region instead of the big city. Housing was much cheaper and with the help of the grant, we could buy or build a bigger home for our expanding family. So, what was planned to be just a three month move became ten years.

I wanted my first two children close together, so when Nathan was seven months old, we decided that we would try again. We successfully conceived and within a week after moving into our newly built home, Merryn was born. Her birth added to my already existing belief and amazement at the perfection of new life produced from marriage and my body, albeit through great pain and fatigue. Nonetheless, it was all worth it. I had purpose in life as a mother and was so happy and content with our perfect pigeon pair.

Life floated along with raising our two children and enjoying living in this regional area of Victoria. During our discussions about how many children we would like, Brian said he didn't want to have an odd number as he felt that one would always be left out. He had come from a family of four children and I had one sibling.

My desire was to have more than two, so we decided that four would be the number. The plan was to have the first two close together, which we had achieved, but I wanted a bit of a gap between number two and three to allow for a time of recovery and management, then a smaller gap to the youngest.

I stopped breastfeeding Merryn when she was eleven months old, and my regular cycle returned. Avoiding pregnancy at my fertile time by using the "Billings method" and condoms appeared to be quite successful in managing the desired spacing of a few years gap before we tried to conceive child number three. But when Merryn had just turned two, I noticed my cycle was different and I felt I was ovulating later. Brian, who did not like to use condoms for longer than was necessary, told me that I wouldn't fall pregnant and to "trust" him. I consented, as I usually did, and allowed him to have his way with me.

Subsequently, I found myself to be pregnant with number three—and a few months later at an ultrasound it became known that we were expecting numbers three *and* four. My desire to have a few years' gap after Merryn became only two years and eight months, and the desired short gap between three and four was definitely going to be short—it ended up being only eighteen minutes!

The pregnancy was fairly routine until about the thirty-week mark when my blood pressure started rising and I spent the rest of the pregnancy in and out of hospital. This was a very stressful time as we had to rely on local friends to help look after Nathan and Merryn while I was in hospital, or ask family to drive the long two-to-three hours from Melbourne to help. The twins, Jared and Rohan, finally arrived only eight days before their due date in January 1987—both healthy and good weights. I suffered intense head and abdominal pain, however, and had an eclamptic fit about an hour after they were born, which resulted in me having to be resuscitated, then I spent the next five hours unconscious. With a battered body that, by the end of my pregnancy, had carried six kilos of babies and survived eclampsia, it took another three weeks to be well enough to venture home and start the mammoth task of nurturing and raising four pre-school children.

As a woman, when you are told to "trust" your partner that you won't fall pregnant, and not only do you fall pregnant but conceive twins, you become much more dismissive of your partner's confidence. Hence, I told Brian not to come near me or touch me as I feared I would get pregnant again—possibly with triplets next time. This, of course, was not welcomed by him. Four children in four years was my physical and emotional limit, so I put up the "no deal" sign.

Then, when the twins were only a few months old, Brian decided to have a vasectomy. I didn't oppose this decision as I was done with pregnancy, and it certainly would protect me from falling pregnant again and take the pressure off being concerned all the time. But once he was given the all clear from the doctor, his concern for my cycle was eliminated.

Being the mother of four very precious children—including the privilege of twin boys—all of whom I will always hold dear to my heart, also brings the enormous financial and physical responsibility of raising them. I wanted to do the best I possibly could so they could eventually go out into the world successfully on their own. Young children need 24/7 care, attention, and support. It does not take much to imagine the workload required to fulfil the many tasks necessary every day to care for two small babies and two pre-schoolers. This is especially difficult when the mother is still recovering from her near-death health scare and the father is at work during the week.

You can imagine how tired I was, and in need of all the sleep I could get when the children were asleep. Brian became resentful of the amount of time I dedicated to taking care of the children, and my need to sleep when I went to bed. His belief that my need for sleep showed a lack of interest in satisfying his sexual desires—which he deemed to be his marital right—was never a deliberate intention by me, but simply the result of having four young children so close together.

So it became his habit to just roll me over in my sleep at any time of the night, get on top of me, move my underwear to the side, then penetrate me and ejaculate. Most of the time when the children were young, I was so tired that I would groggily wake up only enough to realise he was on top of me, and wait for him to get off me so I could go back to sleep. Because I saw these incidents as isolated, I convinced myself they didn't have a lasting impact, which was an easier way to cope than admitting how deeply they affected me. But when these occasions became his normal behaviour, and happened every few weeks, they had a cumulative effect. The feeling of being abused and taken for granted started to severely impact my wellbeing. As these instances increased in frequency, or if I was more fully awake, I would sometimes try to push him off and tell him to get lost. But this became dangerous as he would be impossible to live with the next day. Presumably he desired to punish me with his silent treatment and totally uncooperative behaviour. My way of coping became to pretend to still be asleep and let him have his way with me, otherwise I would suffer his punishment which was unbearable, especially with four children to look after.

His insatiable appetite for sex was impossible to satisfy; he often complained to me that he "would die" if he wasn't able to have sex, and put pressure on me to comply regularly. During that era, people didn't talk about our sexual behaviour with others, so I didn't have anyone else's experience to compare with.

I did wonder, though, about single men who didn't appear to die if they didn't have a partner, but due to my naïvety and having no means to know any better, I believed him. But the more I gave to him when I was awake—usually at least once a week—the more he expected, and the more he would just take from me while I was asleep whenever it suited him. This behaviour of abuse went on for years, greatly impacting my feelings of being used as a mere chattel and compounding my ongoing feelings of unworthiness.

When the twins were six years old, we moved back to Melbourne as the privatisation of the SEC by the Kennett State Government was in full swing and job prospects for advancement were diminishing. Merryn was training with the elite gymnastics squad at the Victorian Institute of Sport and the future education of the children was also part of our decision to return to Melbourne. This meant selling our house and buying another, packing up and moving everything, and finding a new school and job, which was incredibly stressful with four small children in tow.

Moving into a five-bedroom house finally enabled us to give each of the children their own bedroom. The house had an extension upstairs with three bedrooms that all shared a bathroom. Our master bedroom was one of these, and there was not much of a sound barrier across the passage or through the bathroom to two of the children's bedrooms.

One evening, after all the children had gone to bed, Brian attempted to have sex with me but due to his egotistical aggression and total lack of intimate advances, I was unwilling—or more to the point, unable—to respond to him in a positive way. This caused him to become more aggressive and violent. I tried, as quietly as I could so the children would not be disturbed, to hold him off and, in a hushed but forceful tone, communicate to him that he was hurting me and to stop forcing me to comply with his wishes. He kept trying to pin me down to the bed by my wrists as I tried to get free. I was so scared of a repeat of the forceful Tasmanian rape. He finally released my arms and gave up the fight and I fearfully curled up on my side of the bed, wondering where this was all going to end. The silent treatment became his go-to punishment for me as I became less and less able to respond to his advances. But I was determined to keep the vow I had made to myself after the honeymoon and continued to bow to his advances, using *fawning* (when an individual tries to avoid or minimise distress or danger by pleasing and appeasing the threat) on numerous occasions to just keep the peace, even though it was becoming harder and harder for me to relax and give myself to him. The rapes in my sleep were still occuring. The default scenario became that he would expect his "needs" to be met every weekend.

At no time in our intimate relationship did he ever try to be a compassionate, loving partner and enable me to enjoy the intimacy that a woman should expect from a considerate partner. It was all one way for him.

While visiting a girlfriend (whose husband was a close friend of Brian's), during a school holiday catch-up with our children, I broke down in tears from the pressure of the abuse, rapes, lack of sleep, silent treatment, and fear. She was shocked by my sudden out-of-the-blue breakdown. And so was I. I was so embarrassed. What happened in the bedroom, I felt, should stay in the bedroom. However, I also felt obliged to tell her what was wrong with me. The words just tumbled out and she heard everything I was experiencing. Her immediate response was that his behaviour was not normal; no abuse was normal. I felt relieved that I had finally told someone but also embarrassed by my predicament and the disclosure of my husband's behaviour. A submissive wife didn't do that, did she? She didn't blab about her husband.

Later, I felt so remorseful for telling my secret that I told her everything was fine, and that I would work it out and was okay. I couldn't cope with someone knowing about my intimate issues. It was incredibly embarrassing.

The years tumbled on and I continued to make every effort to quell the tension between us and meet his needs. But it became harder and harder to relax, and my ability to get a good night's sleep diminished significantly. Brian also started to wear hearing aids, so I had to make sure I had his attention before I could speak to him.

Organising life around the activities of four late primary and early secondary-aged children was hectic. His punishment was to ignore me and pretend to not hear me, but I was never sure if he hadn't heard me or if he was deliberately using passive-aggressive behaviour. Not knowing which it was, my inflection would become frustrated and my volume would increase as I repeated my request for his attention. This would be repeated several times until he would scream at me that he wasn't going to talk to me because I was shouting at him. Our household was a total disaster.

Imagining life to be something it wasn't was my only mechanism to be able to function. But Brian's destructive behaviour never let up. His ability to roll me over in my sleep became impossible as I began to wake up and push him away; I just couldn't do it anymore. On a number of occasions, he would masturbate against my body and smear my upper leg with his semen. Fear would run through my body during the night as, on many occasions, I would wake up to a gently rocking bed as he masturbated until he ejaculated.

He gave up touching me, stating I was deliberately depriving him of his marital rights. My response was that I needed to be loved and cherished for who I was as his wife and not for what he could get from me. He wasn't loving me at all. His reply was that he wanted to love me, but I was pushing him away. Somehow in his language "love" was spelt "S. E. X."

Spending countless wakeful nights pretending to be asleep, I often witnessed him climb out of bed and masturbate on the floor. Waking up at around 3 am one morning, I found the bed empty and no presence of him in the room or bathroom, so I ventured downstairs. The rumpus room light shone from under the closed door and the soft sound of the TV could be heard as I approached the door. Instead of slowly opening the door, thereby alerting him of my presence, I burst into the room and was confronted with the sight of him sitting on the couch with his erect penis raised into the air as he watched a movie on the TV. In shock I pleaded with him to show me respect as his wife and to stop his selfish and insensitive behaviour which was conveying to me that I did not matter. His response was that I did not need to know what he got up to and it was none of my business what he did to himself since I was depriving him of his marital rights. I replied that a marriage is not built on control, coercion, and self-interest. It must be built on mutual love, respect, and wellbeing for each other, and it did matter what he was up to as it showed no love, respect, or consideration for my wellbeing. Furthermore, I said I was not deliberately depriving him but was frozen in an inability to respond to him due to years of his coercion, manipulation, and abuse without any concern for my feelings or welfare. He told me to "sort myself out." I went back to bed alone, and cried.

In an effort to give the children some enjoyable life experiences, we made plans to visit the theme parks on Queensland's Gold Coast during the September school holidays. We flew to Coolangatta and booked coaches to travel between our apartment in Surfers Paradise and the theme parks. Giving them all a memorable trip was my aim, and I worked hard to produce delicious meals and a relaxing environment, all while feeling increasingly depressed and hopeless.

One free afternoon, we stayed in our apartment and the children watched a movie in the lounge room. While I was trying to relax by reading on the bed, Brian approached me for sex and, as my aim had been to give everyone a great time, I relented and allowed him to have what he wanted. Feeling used and totally devoid from engaging with him, I just wanted to escape his coercion and the life that surrounded me.

Glancing outside, I noticed that there was no fly screen on the open nineteenth floor apartment window. That feeling of despair, worthlessness, and hopelessness overwhelmed me and escaping from Brian became paramount. What I had been resisting for years overtook me and I started to move to the window, intending to fly through the air and escape his clutches. My rational decision-making left my awareness for a split second, until a picture of my four precious children entered my consciousness and I checked my movement.

Brian was getting dressed at the end of the bed and had no idea what had transpired over those few seconds of my life. When I looked at him, his face appeared to me like a monster who wanted to devour their prey, not a supposed "loving husband" who had just had sex with his beloved wife. I remember saying that his face was contorted and his appearance seemed possessed by evil. I told him that he had lost all control of his desires and I couldn't go on like this, that we needed help to save our family. Quickly shaking his head, as if to remove the appearance I had described, he, for the first time ever, admitted to being out of control sexually and said that we probably did need some professional support. We agreed to seek help from our Pastor and his wife when we returned to Melbourne. The first glimmer of hope!

After our holiday we organised that meeting with the Pastor, and during it we both described what was going on in our relationship. He was quite shocked at our revelations and asked how I was coping. I stated I wasn't, that I was very depressed, had become suicidal, and that I was incredibly concerned for the welfare of the children. He suggested I spend some time talking through my pain with another counsellor, and that Brian should have sessions with them to work through his issues.

At last, some progress was being made. We made the decision to tell our families that we were struggling in our relationship, but were hopeful that in receiving counselling, we would be able to rescue our marriage.

...break me
...make me
...goal
...stronger
...longer
...my soul

4

"Mum, He's My Dad"

From Merryn's Perspective

"Life doesn't come with a manual; it comes with a mother."
—Author Unknown.

Author's Note: *The following chapter is written from the perspective of my daughter, whose story and reflections form a deeply personal part of this book, in the hope it will provide some balance from a child's viewpoint. It was written with her full knowledge and explicit permission, following her careful review of the content. These experiences are shared here with her blessing, with the mutual desire that our mother–daughter healing process may resonate with and support others on similar paths.*

MY EARLIEST COMFORTING MEMORY is of curling up on my mother's lap, sucking my thumb as she cuddled me. Feeling secure, I sensed that her breathing was much slower than mine and I tried to regulate my breathing to match hers, to feel at one with her. Her rings fascinated me, and I loved to fiddle with them and turn them around on her fingers. It was soothing to be close to my mother. Having three brothers, though, meant we had to share our time on her comforting lap. Nathan was sixteen months older than me, and the twins, Jared and Rohan, were two years and eight months younger. I don't remember the time of the twins' birth at all, as I was only two years old, but I do recall being told that it was a stressful time for us as a family because Mum was in hospital for quite a while. From the beginning, my recollections have always involved my three brothers and a busy household.

Gymnastics was a big part of my life from when I was five years old. When I was eight, I was selected to join the International Victorian Elite Squad, which was one of the contributing factors for my family moving back to Melbourne from the Latrobe Valley where my father had been working for the SEC. After one year I moved over to a National Club. We lived in a two-storey house with three bedrooms upstairs and two downstairs. My parents' bedroom was upstairs with a walk-through wardrobe to a shared bathroom and toilet. My bedroom was across the passage from the bathroom, so it was quite easy for me to hear noise from my parents' bedroom, even with the door closed, as the sound carried through the wardrobe and bathroom. On many occasions I heard my mother being upset with my father, but I couldn't hear any response or retaliation from him. My mother was often very angry with my father, and as a nine-year-old girl I was scared that my mother would be dead in the morning, that my father would kill her due to her treatment toward him. I found it hard to sleep and cried a lot.

After a few years, my parents decided to move to a new house that was closer to our school. My mother often seemed upset with my father and would yell at him; she yelled and screamed at us kids as well. Thankfully, gymnastics enabled me to be out of the house a lot. Most of the time my mother drove me, and she came to all my competitions while my father stayed home with my brothers.

Holidays were great experiences and we visited numerous places. During our trip to the Gold Coast when I was fourteen, we had great fun on the rides and activities at the theme parks. Mum usually waited at the rides with our stuff and only occasionally got involved. She seemed incredibly sad and did not talk much with Dad. Coming home, we had to change flights in Sydney and Dad left his jumper in the overhead locker. Mum realised he didn't have it as we walked to the gate for our connecting flight. She was so angry with him, which was a regular occurrence for her. I was so embarrassed by her reaction. She made him ask a flight attendant if they were able to retrieve it, which they managed to do. It was a very quiet flight home after that because we were all too scared to talk.

Not long before my parents separated, we went to Ulladulla for Easter with our aunt (Dad's sister), uncle, cousins, and other families who were friendly with them. It was a long drive and my siblings and I became bored. At one point while Mum was driving, Dad hurt Nathan's finger by reaching back from the front seat and twisting it around. It was so bruised it turned black. I could tell Mum was upset with Dad, but she seemed to bottle it all in on this occasion. She tried to give us an enjoyable holiday, but I feared my parents.

Gymnastics remained a huge distraction in my life, but I started to have many injuries and eventually had to give it up. This was so disappointing as I loved it, and it helped me be very disciplined in the use of my time. My mother suggested I try coaching, so we asked at the local YMCA centre if I could volunteer to gain experience by working with a coach, which they were happy for me to do. If I could not do gymnastics anymore, at least I could stay involved with it, and I loved working with the little kids.

My parents, I think, tried to get some help to save their marriage but I wasn't surprised when they told us they were separating. Dad left and rented a house not far away. I felt like it was my responsibility to comfort my mother to prevent her from killing herself as I could tell she was very depressed. She would tell me awful things about my father and what he had done to her, but I didn't want to hear it or believe it. Basically, she wanted me to disown my father—and that was never going to happen. One of the things she said was that my father didn't deserve to walk me down the aisle when I got married. I told her that that would be my decision, not hers. As I was only fifteen when my parents separated, I didn't need to face that issue, but I already knew what I wanted.

The four of us children were taken to a counselling place where—individually and as a group—we were asked how we felt about our parents separating. I remember being asked to draw pictures to express my emotions. It was an incredibly stressful time and I cried a lot. As we were old enough to make the decision ourselves, we were each asked which parent we would like to live with. Independently of each other, we all chose to live with our mother, as she was the one that did nearly all the work in looking after us, but I would have preferred to not have had to make the decision as I think my mother thought that I was taking her side, which I wasn't. The decision just had to be made as to what was best for us at that time.

Struggling financially, my mother thought it a good idea for me to get my first job so I could have my own money. Nathan was already working at McDonalds at the time. After taking my resume into various shops at our local shopping centre, I was so excited to be offered a few shifts a week at a chemist. This was a great experience for me, and soon afterwards, I was also offered a gymnastics coaching job after school. So between the two jobs, I worked a few hours every day after school and most Saturdays for about six years while completing secondary school and studying nursing. Being away from home suited me just fine as it meant I didn't have to be around my dependent mother.

Our family home was sold, and my mother built a new house about nine kilometres from our home and school. It took about fifteen minutes to drive there instead of being able to walk to school as we did before. The move happened when I was in Year Eleven, Nathan was Year Twelve, and the twins were in Year Eight. It was such a big upheaval. This was the fourth house I had lived in so far in my life. Soon after we moved, I did my debutante with school and relished the whole experience. I was delighted to have my dress made, attend the dance lessons, ride in a limousine with my girlfriends, and enjoy the night of the debutante ball. The spoiler, though, was that I became really upset with my mother when she made me arrive late to the rehearsal at Rembrandts, and she refused to sit at the same table as my father and his family which meant we had to book two different tables. What was supposed to be a girl's highlight experience of growing up with her friends was marred by my parents' standoff.

Upon completing Year Twelve, I was accepted into the nursing course I had applied for at Monash University. Thankfully, I was able to save up enough money to buy my own car. It was incredibly exciting to get my driver's license and become independent from my mother; no longer relying on her, I could come and go as I pleased. My brothers and I spent many Sundays with our father for lunch and enjoyed the occasional gathering with his family. Although my nursing course was enjoyable, after about two years I was struggling to cope with being at home, so when a girlfriend suggested I do a Bible Study course as a gap year, as she had done, I investigated it further and decided it was worth my while to give it a go.

The church I was still attending with my family was running the course at another centre about thirty minutes' drive from home. It involved living with a family who became my spiritual parents for the year and helped guide me along on my spiritual journey. The group included twelve young people, who each had a mentor as well as their spiritual parents, and involved Bible study, community work which included going into secondary schools, team building sessions, learning leadership skills, and attending church on Sundays. Once a month I returned to my own church to stay connected with the people there. I had to give up my jobs, which was sad, but I was able to receive Austudy payments from Centrelink that covered the costs of my course, running my car, and necessary living expenses. It was so good to escape from home and be away from my mother. Nathan had gone overseas this same year, and the twins were doing Year Twelve.

During the course I was encouraged to deal with issues I was having in my life, and during counselling was able to talk these through and discuss my feelings about the issues with my parents. They were adamant that I needed to have more respect for my dad and improve my relationship with him. As for Mum, I shared that as her only daughter, I sensed her dependence on me immensely and felt the responsibility for her continued existence. I made them aware that her behaviour included frequently yelling at us kids, as she had also done to my dad when they were still together. I also shared how she had told me about bad things Dad had done to her, and that she didn't believe he deserved to walk me down the aisle at my wedding. Their response was that they believed my mum was co-dependent on me and suggested that I work on my relationship with my dad without the influence from my mum. They also said she needed to respect my decisions. I realised that I needed to exercise stronger boundaries in our relationship and that when I spoke to her, Dad was off limits. Due to the busyness of the course, I hardly saw my mother during this year.

The course taught me so much about myself and I grew up a lot while gaining many great friendships and achieving independence. But even though I felt refreshed and ready to return to university for the final year of my nursing degree, I still had to move back home with my mother. After living away from home for this time, my perspective had changed, and on my return, I did feel that my mother struggled with my changed attitude towards her.

I tried to get some work back at the chemist and the gymnastics club, but I had long placements in my final year and it wasn't practical to have set shifts at work that I wouldn't be able to honour. As a result, I didn't have any income other than the basic Austudy. My mother wanted me to pay board, but I told her I didn't have enough as I needed to run my car and pay for other living expenses.

My father married again and I think my mother found this hard to cope with, especially when Nathan returned from overseas and went to live with them a few months after their wedding.

My mother suffered from ongoing headaches, so she decided to move away from the electric substation that was right near her bedroom wall. She planned on building two units, to live in one and sell the other, but this meant selling the house to get access to the equity, meaning she would need to rent a property during the construction period. A four-bedroom house was required to fit the twins and me, which was more expensive and harder to find than a three-bedroom house. Mum and I were having a hard time living together because the year away had changed my perspective. I found it difficult to cope with her stressful life and we both struggled with the new boundaries I had set. After a couple of months, my dad and his wife said I could live with them.

This was different to living with Mum. It was a healing and positive time and I was able to sort out a lot of the issues I had with him during the eighteen months I lived there. On finishing my degree, I was fortunate to land a rewarding job in the Paediatric Ward at Monash Hospital, Clayton. Mum rented a house and both the twins went to live with her.

During this time, I was without a car for four weeks, so I lived with Mum while working at Monash Hospital. Jared had gone to housesit for a friend while he was overseas, so there was room for me at Mum's which was only a few kilometres away from Monash Hospital. If I had an early shift, I was able to ride my scooter to work and back to Mum's again, but if I had an afternoon shift it was dark by the time I finished, and Mum would come and pick me up, which I appreciated. She seemed to be a bit happier and easier to get on with, which made it okay to live with her again for a short time. Once I got my car back, I returned to live with Dad.

Then Nathan and his girlfriend got engaged; as the only girl in the family, gaining a sister-in-law was very exciting. Both our parents attended their engagement party, but Rohan rang the following Monday to tell me that Mum was extremely upset. Dad had warned him that Mum would be receiving a letter from him after the party—and that she may be upset when she read it—but he didn't tell Rohan what it was about. I told him to not get involved as it was about time that Mum and Dad sorted out their own differences and it was none of our business. Rohan had also told me that Dad was suggesting he live with them to get away from our mother as she was "dangerous, very destructive, and manipulative." I didn't want to get involved anymore; I'd had enough of the bickering.

The next family occasion was the twins' twenty-first birthday, and they decided to celebrate at Dad's house as they had a large rumpus/entertainment room. The issue was that Dad and his wife had decided that Mum was too dangerous and wouldn't be welcome to come to their house. Mum had told the twins that she wouldn't be able to come if they held their party there, as our father had made it very clear to her that she was not welcome in their home. But she also understood that the twins really didn't have any other option due to cost, so she just said she couldn't be there.

I remember Rohan having a huge argument with Dad and his wife, accusing them of not co-operating to enable our parents to be civil to each other, which was making it very hard for us. He said he didn't care what Dad and his wife thought of our mother, and that he and Jared wanted her at their twenty-first party. I didn't want to get involved. When they saw how angry Rohan was, they gave in, rang Mum, and invited her to come. She agreed on the grounds she would be welcomed, and Dad reluctantly guaranteed that she would. The party happened and all went well. Thank goodness!

Nathan's wedding followed a few months later and his fiancée invited Mum and me to the house where she was getting dressed; it was a thoughtful gesture to include us in this part of the celebration and included photos with all the girls and her family. At the church, Mum and I moved down to the front, then Nathan reminded me that he had intended to walk Mum and his future mother-in-law down the aisle to their seats, but I had forgotten to tell her. Mum had a quick chat with Nathan, then sat in the front row where the mother of the groom usually sits. Dad's wife was already there and looked cross with Mum, gesturing to her to move further down the seat where my grandparents were already seated. My father, who had been chatting with Nathan's groomsmen, returned to find Mum sitting where he had been sitting. He and his wife chatted and didn't look happy, and they had to move down the seat to fit Dad in while I sat with relatives in the row behind. Even with all this going on, both the wedding ceremony and the reception on the Yarra River were great celebrations.

Around this time, I started courting Phil, who I met through mentoring participants in the Bible Study course. We were both supported by our respective spiritual parents. He was living nearby so I decided that it was a good idea to venture out on my own and move into a shared house with others from the church. Six months later he delivered a romantic proposal to me at the Rhododendron Gardens in the Dandenong Ranges and had secretly organised for our families to be present for a picnic lunch so we could surprise them with our exciting news. I was so happy. Our engagement party was at Dad's house and Mum came without any of the dramas of the twins' twenty-first birthday party.

Hesitantly, I asked Mum if I could come to her place (she had moved into her completed unit and had sold the other one) to use her sewing machine. She seemed happy for me to come around, and we had dinner together as well. Her demeanour was a lot happier and we refrained from mentioning Dad and his wife at all. Once I was engaged, Phil moved in with his parents to save money. We thought it better for me to conserve spending as well, so I asked Mum if I could move into the new unit with her as it was in a good location for me to get to work at Monash Hospital. Eliminating financial issues, I was prepared to cover costs of utilities and food.

I mentioned to her that I had asked Dad to walk me down the aisle and said that if she wasn't comfortable with my decision, it was up to her if she came or not. There was no further comment from her, and she seemed to just accept it. I appreciated the time that we shared to talk through wedding plans and work together to organise my special day. Mum sewed the two flower girls' dresses and they turned out just the way I wanted. She also made the bridal party fur capes to keep us warm, which were much appreciated on the cool winter's day of our wedding. Overall, it was pleasurable being around my mother, but we avoided touching on the pressure points that existed between us.

Even though I was living with Mum again when I

was getting married, I wanted to spend the night before my wedding at Dad's as there was room for me to have my bridesmaids stay with me. It was a first-class venue for getting ready and having our hair and makeup done together. This meant that it became another occasion that Mum had to be allowed to come to Dad's house, which they weren't happy about, but really, they had no choice. Knowing how I felt about the situation, I think Mum wanted my special day to go without a hitch and she worked extremely hard to enable that to happen, and I was more interested in enjoying the moment than worrying about how she was coping.

The day flowed well, as I had hoped, and along with my grandparents, Mum and Dad sat at the parents' table, albeit on opposite sides. Rohan was recruited to dance with Mum after the bridal waltz as I knew she would feel hurt to be left with no one to dance with after the "Dad and Daughter dance" when Dad went to dance with his wife.

Shortly after our wedding, Mum announced that she was seeing someone she had met at university where she was studying theology. The four of us were thrilled for her as we did want to see her happy. Mum and Ted got engaged a few months later with a wedding to follow a few months after that. Originally Mum hadn't asked me to be her Matron of Honour, but when I asked her why she hadn't asked me, she said she didn't think I would want to. I told her I would relish the opportunity to help, and she asked me immediately if I would like to be part of her bridal party. She had already asked a friend she had made from her new church, and together we supported Mum. Ted had a few granddaughters who were gorgeous flower girls, and their wedding was a joyous day. I felt some relief that Mum had someone to share life with, and that she would be less dependent on us.

About six months later we shared our exciting news that we were expecting our first child. Knowing how excited Mum would be, we organised a family dinner with Mum, Ted, and my grandparents to break the news to them. Mum was over the moon. Over the next few months, I did enjoy sharing my baby plans with Mum and she helped pick up a cot and baby cradle that I purchased second-hand. She enjoyed being involved by coming on shopping trips and witnessing my ultrasound to find out the gender. A little girl!

I invited her to the birth, in one way to support Phil but also to share with her the birth of her grandchild. It was a harrowing labour where both Phil and I valued that added support. Once we were home, we sent out an SOS call to Mum to help buy more mop-up cloths as our little girl was a real spewer.

Mum was around often and helped with the household chores and all the usual activities with her granddaughter. So, when I planned to go back to work for two shifts a fortnight, Mum was the go-to babysitter one day a week. Mum seemed to relish the time with her granddaughter, and my daughter was always happy to go with her Grandma. Mum did this until I went on maternity leave again when expecting our second child. She would have been at the baby's birth but it was too quick and she missed it, although she was there soon after. When I came home, Mum, again, helped with chores and was heavily involved with both the girls, and bonded well with number two. I had post-natal depression and some feeding issues after giving birth to her and it was supportive to be able to ring Mum when I needed; these are the times you need your mum at the other end of the phone and by your side. She was caring and helped me get through that difficult time. She then babysat the girls when I returned to work one day a week, before falling pregnant again with child number three.

By this stage we had a three-year-old and our second was just over twelve months old. The school that we intended to send the girls to (the same school that I had attended) ran an activity group for pre-schoolers. Although it was great, I found it exceedingly difficult to attend as each child needed one-on-one attention, so I asked Mum if she would help. She joined us and thoroughly enjoyed being involved with the girls, so when number three arrived, between us we looked after the three of them. Afterwards, Mum would usually come home with us and help me with the housework, shopping, cleaning, washing, and cooking us a meal. This arrangement continued for the next five years as each of the girls grew and headed off to school.

During our last year at *Art Place*, while the older two were at school I received a phone call from my stepmother. In total shock she told me that my father had received a phone call out of the blue from the police and had been summoned to attend an interview to answer questions relating to the alleged sexual abuse and rape of my mother. I couldn't believe what I was hearing.

Why on earth was she doing this? And why now?

My stepmother was furious and so was I.

What was wrong with my mother to do this after all this time?

I told my stepmother I would call Mum and chastise her. I made that phone call and asked my mother if she had anything to tell me. My mother's response was that I had phoned her, so I angrily confronted her, "Mum! What do you think you are doing? What about forgiveness? What good will come of going to the police? He's my dad!"

It was over two years before I spoke to my mother again.

...wise
... pain
...price
...gained
...anything

5

Breaking The Silence

"There are so many predators in the world, but silence itself may be chief among them. It is deadly. When it comes to recovery, silence is the knife edge between illness and health. Between dignity and indignity. For some, between life and death."
—Lucia Osborne-Crowley, *I Choose Elena*

So, what do we do to try and find a way to heal a person's ailing mental health from the destructiveness of sexual abuse? The social expectations of "suck it up" or "just get on with life" have been the solutions for past generations, and that has worked—hasn't it?

As a society there was no pressure for anything to be exposed as no-one wanted to listen, or cared to understand about the effects on mental health. Perpetrators didn't need to admit to their destructive behaviour as no-one challenged them to be held to account, and women and other victims suffered in silence. Divorce was difficult to obtain in Australia until the no-fault system came into law in 1976, and women weren't allowed to work when married in the Commonwealth public service before 1966. So they were dependent on their husbands for financial support for themselves and their children. This gender inequality resulted in many abused women taking their agony to the grave. So, has this approach been a successful solution? I do not think so! I feel so, so sorry for those who endured in silence. They never had a chance to speak of their pain, to be heard, nor to experience justice and healing.

Whatever the abuse suffered by people, whether sexual or physical violence, a criminal offence, parental negligence, family abuse, or bullying in the school yard, it is everyone's individual story. No one outcome is the same as another. There are many resulting effects on people's lives and those around them, just as there are so many different traumas that have been suffered.

Once I revealed my secret, I heard a few repeated comments from people in my community. For example, I was told that all I needed to do was to forgive, and that would resolve all my issues. But even though I forgave over and over again, this didn't work. Then others would put the blame back on me as being the problem; I was the one who was not able to recover some semblance of a normal disposition. I had forgiven, and I was fighting to be "normal," but I realised there was more needed than just to "forgive and move on." There are many more aspects to the healing process. All this just added to my frustration, pain, and alienation.

If forgiveness works for you, and you are able to have a good relationship with the abuser and they are still a part of your life, then that is great for you. Or if the passage of time has healed your trauma and it is no longer a defining element in your life, then again that is so, so good and pleasing to hear. But what of the many people who have not been healed by time, or those who continue to experience pain even after forgiving the perpetrator over, and over, and over again? Or when a person's life remains a burden, or they lack a fulfilling existence, and that burden overflows to affect their family and the precious relationships around them? There must be other ways to recover and achieve healing!

Counselling with a professional has its place, even just to talk through the trauma and learn strategies to minimise the impact of reliving events and remove the hold that abusers can have. Rapid Eye Movement techniques, deep breathing, crossing one's arms over and tapping your hands on your shoulders, shrinking the perpetrator into a small square shape and putting them—figuratively—in some distant place, can all assist to lessen the hold of the trauma.

I have been to many counsellors over the years. Most did not even hone-in on the trauma I have experienced but only tried to put out spot fires in my immediate life.

One of the biggest changes that has helped me to start the road to recovery has been reading Lucia Osborne-Crowley's book, *I Choose Elena*. I saw her being interviewed on the ABC show, *The Drum*, where she shared about her sexual abuse experience and I immediately knew I needed to read her story. A high achieving gymnast heading for Olympic standard competition, she was cruelly stopped in her tracks when she was violently assaulted and raped at the age of fifteen. This resulted in health issues that continued to plague her body for years afterwards. But that violent event wasn't the start of her demise; it was the final catalyst. It wasn't until one day, about ten years later, while shopping at a supermarket of all places, that she started to join the dots of her memories. She writes:

Memories of a man in our gymnastics community who sexually abused me as a child. A man I adored. A man I admired. A man who had hurt me, again and again and again and again. Of course I already knew this.

The part of me that froze in that moment was full of every memory of inappropriate contact he made with me; full of frozen moments during massages that went too far; frozen moments during cuddles that didn't feel right. He had crossed many boundaries that I had pretended to ignore but in this moment, I no longer could. He had groomed me for years; a fact I knew in my body, in my muscles, but had never accepted in my mind.

In that moment, it felt as though the whole world would collapse. Instead, I did. I fell to the floor and sat there, frozen, crying, confused, in the middle of the condiments aisle. *(Osborne-Crowley 2020, 109–10.)*

She had finally joined the dots of shame to understand that as a young gymnast she had been a victim, an easy target, vulnerable to trauma, and groomed to respond with a freeze response so her coach could continue his subtle, damaging perpetration. So at fifteen, when an unknown random male predator made his move on her, she allowed him to take her by the hand and lead her away to a secluded place. Another fifteen year old, not similarly groomed, potentially would have screamed the place down, gone into flight mode, and escaped. It's like the well-known analogy of the frog in boiling water: If a frog is dropped into boiling water, it will immediately jump out to survive. But if it's placed in tepid water that is slowly brought to the boil, it won't perceive the danger and will be boiled alive. In the same way, we can become desensitised to escalating harm, unaware of the need to escape until it's too late. Shame had kept Osborne-Crowley silent about the childhood abuse, just as it did the assault and rape when she was fifteen. Until it was almost too late.

The name *I Choose Elena* comes from the *Neapolitan* series of books written by Elena Ferrante, where she tells the story of two young women, Elena and Lila, who were best friends and confidantes while growing up in Naples in the 1950s and 60s. When Elena, the narrator, starts the book at the end of her story by describing the disappearance of Lila, she is not surprised to learn that Lila has gone missing. Elena tells her readers that Lila had always wanted to become invisible. Lila had suffered much trauma as a child and had confided to Elena that she wanted to vanish with no trace to be found. Osborne-Crowley writes:

> Any person who has moved through the world with the body of a woman will know what it feels like to wish to be invisible. In the end, Lila never escapes this feeling. She finds a way to disappear. I don't blame her. Overcoming this feeling is one of the hardest lessons a woman can learn. It is an ongoing act of survival. *(Osborne-Crowley 2020, 9).*

Osborne-Crowley then goes on to tell her story of trauma and the nearly fatal destruction that this has had on her body and her life. She chose to be like Elena, who admitted to her own traumatic life but continued to face up to and live through her challenges. She remained visible. This meant recording her story, in contrast to Lila who wanted to keep her traumatic story under wraps, and not face her challenges but slip further and further away from people until she completely disappeared without a trace. No one knew where she had gone.

Osborne-Crowley had kept her story of trauma silent and became invisible by disengaging from people and allowing herself to be repeatedly abused by men who took advantage of her. I connected with her story and realised I had also been invisible and hidden my grief. By going to the police, I had started to reveal my story. But then I suffered because my children were not coping with the exposure of their father's bad behaviour toward their mother. They stopped contacting me, which made me feel even more invisible and caused me to suffer even more severe mental health problems.

Isolating in lockdowns during the COVID-19 pandemic only reinforced the situation of lack of face-to-face contact with my family. This was not the ideal time to combat, and overcome, my desire to be invisible. It was much easier to hide away in my house and not have to speak to anybody. My son, Nathan, who was living in Hong Kong as a teacher, made the suggestion via a WhatsApp family group of holding a family Zoom meeting. At that time, I was only reading comments in the group chat and never replied because their father was also in the group. Of course, I was being invisible and, naturally, we don't comment when we are invisible. There was no way my depressed mental health would enable me to be on the same Zoom as him and the children, who had wanted to keep their distance from me for quite some time. According to me, this was a naïve and thoughtless suggestion for them to make. In ordinary family circumstances though, this would have been a good idea—especially during a prolonged time of lockdowns and isolation—that would be beneficial for family connection.

This incident was the straw that broke the camel's back and sent me further to the depths of depression, causing me to experience a complete physical shutdown. I can fully empathise with people actually ending their lives. There is this pull that part of you wants to just stop the pain and end it all as it is too hard to fathom any hope or discern a positive outcome. Then there is the other part that wants to live but be invisible to those around you and forget the destructiveness you are experiencing. It was only through the support of Ted emailing my children to explain my reaction to the suggested Zoom meeting, that they started to have some in-depth understanding as to the seriousness of my mental health.

While I was in this highly depressed state, my father rang to have a chat and catch me up with what had been going on with him and Mum. When you want to be invisible, you hide how you are really feeling from the people you love, but when the depths of depression become so overwhelming, the pain takes over. My father only had to mention my children and I couldn't cope with it any longer. I overflowed with pain and the feelings of shame and anger, and had to hang up the phone. Crying, I asked Ted to ring my father back and tell him what was going on and why I couldn't talk to anyone at that moment.

The next afternoon, I walked down to our beach as we were experiencing a king tide with a strong south-westerly wind and swell which caused the waves to crash into the sand bank along our coastline. This was worth seeing and quite a good way for me to distance myself from the despair of life and, instead, be surrounded by the power of creation. After a king tide comes a king low tide, so early on Easter Sunday morning, I put on warm clothes and kayak shoes, rolled-up my trousers, and walked out on the rocks and sand to find solace for my troubled soul. Before this, I had never taken much interest in the tide being so low, but this time I walked on rocks and sand that I was sure were rarely left uncovered by the seawater, and probably had not been walked upon or observed often.

What was usually hidden under the water was revealed to the daylight and, more significantly, to me.

While I stood there, watching as the sea trickled out over sand and past the end of the rocks with the still falling tide, I had an epiphany of my life, just as Osborne-Crowley encountered in the supermarket. Painful experiences in my childhood that I had kept hidden and covered up, and had thought were gone for good, were now glaringly exposed to me, just as the sand and rocks were exposed by the king low tide. The ramifications of these experiences had resulted in my troubled life. I think my "felt sense" was connecting with the awe of my surroundings as my body was inhaling and absorbing the wonder of the scene.

My life experiences as a small girl primarily involved feeling insecure. My mother did not cope well, which she expressed by losing control, crying and screaming, throwing things, shutting me in my bedroom, and on many occasions, simply disappearing and spending hours in her bedroom. I remember never being angry about this and grew up understanding that my mother couldn't help her behaviour. It was just who she was. It wasn't until I was twelve years old that she was finally diagnosed with the postnatal depression that she had suffered since my older sister was born and for which she had received no assistance or treatment. I have always loved my mother, and even as a small child I remember trying to comfort her by hugging her when I could.

The other revelation I recalled on the rocks was the treatment I received from my maternal grandmother. I felt I had previously dealt with the effects of her behaviour, but here I was again reliving her abuse. Abuse that I had felt wasn't as bad as other people had had to put up with, so I downplayed its impact on me. But now, as an adult, I was living through the mental and emotional effects I had suffered as an insecure little girl. No matter how hard I tried to please her, she constantly put me down, telling me that I couldn't do anything right, that I was an absolute failure, and that I would come to nothing. Then there were the endless comparisons she made between my older sister and me, saying in front of me that my sister did everything the right way and blatantly stating that I did everything the wrong way. She would also hit me if I handed her a piece of cake or toast because I had touched and contaminated it. She died when I was twelve. My sister was bequeathed quite a few of her items and my mother gave me a lovely set of books and a sewing machine, saying they were from my grandmother. But later, when I was a young adult, my mother told me they had come from her, not my grandmother, because my mum was upset that I had not been left anything. My sister never capitalised on this attention and, at the time, was seemingly unaware of our grandmother's strange behaviour and favouritism.

While I sat on the rocks, my mind continued to flash back and reveal many childhood images of instances that had caused me trauma. One revelation was about starting secondary school. I suffered from "school refusal" and on many occasions, I would stop on my way to school, turn around, and go back home because I was unable to cope with the anxiety of the impending day. If I made it to school, I spent much of the time quietly crying in class, struggling to cope with my surroundings and enduring spiteful bullying to which I had no recourse. Additional to this school trauma, I struggled with a learning disability and dyslexia, which added to my insecurities and difficulty in coping with a highly competitive peer pressure environment during my teen years.

Just as Osborne-Crowley connected her gymnastics experience with the violent rape, out on those rocks and sand I started to join the dots of my traumatic life experiences; I felt so vulnerable amidst the wonderful beauty of Mother Nature. And just as Osborne-Crowley found answers to her revelations, I also felt there had to be meaning in so much being revealed to me—for me to find answers to be able to move forward successfully in my life. After my grandmother died, I had made a vow that I would prove her wrong, that I wasn't a failure, and that I would succeed in my life. I met a man, the son of a clergyman, and fell in love. So there was my chance to prove I was normal and not a failure. My plan was to be the perfect wife, have lots of perfect children in a perfect house that I would manage perfectly, and prove to her that I was nothing like she had made me out to be. I would live happily ever after, unaffected, successful, and content with my life. But this was not to be.

The frog should have jumped out of the slowly warming water well before she did, but I froze due to embarrassment, immaturity, stupidity, and my vow to myself. In my way of thinking, all I could do was stay with him, otherwise I would be a failure, just as my grandmother had said I would be. The vow to myself became extended to include that I would stay with Brian and do whatever I had to do to make the marriage work—that was what women did, I had thought. Suffering in silence, I didn't talk to anyone or try to get any help. Later, I worked out the rapes would have happened around sixty times during the remaining twelve years of our marriage. At different times, I would wake up and go into a frozen state. There were occasions that I did push him away, but I was always mindful of him violently raping me again. He would also revert to his ever-growing method of punishment toward me with his passive-aggressive behaviour which was demoralising and divisive and totally unproductive in managing the task of looking after a family together. I just kept letting him do it to me as I was too scared to say no. The frog stayed in the ever-warming water, too frozen to move.

All through this time I was experiencing extreme premenstrual tension and agonising period pain. My moods would swing violently over the course of a month, making normal home activities exceedingly stressful, especially with very active children. But life had to go on. I continued to struggle to be the perfect mother and wife I needed to be without asking for help to fulfil my vow. But I wasn't coping. My attempts to ask Brian and the children for support to keep the housework under control hadn't worked, but I didn't know what else to do. Most of the time Brian would just ignore me. There wasn't much co-operation from him, and the children were just being children. I reverted to being like my own mother, shouting and screaming. The more I wasn't heard and understood, the more I shouted and screamed to try and manage the workload.

As the tide started to slowly return, I wandered back along the beach with my mind full of visions. Then I sat on the sand dune, gazed out across the crystal-clear water, and pondered. I saw myself trying desperately to cope, doing nearly all the housework, and driving the children to and from their various activities by myself. My ambition to be that perfect wife and mother had been a totally unrealistic ideal, and even though I was totally aware of who I had become, I was now staring at the whole picture. I had become just like my mother, who hadn't coped, and I had learnt to behave in the same way. I had allowed Brian to control me because I didn't think I was good enough to be treated any other way. My grandmother had cemented in my mind that I wasn't worthy to be loved as a treasured wife and mother, and so I allowed continual sexual and emotional abuse to rule, causing me continual anxiety and deep depression. I received the insight that what happens to us as innocent children can have lifelong ramifications that can be passed down the generations. Sadly, I was part of that continuing generational chain.

My thoughts moved on to the unnerving catalyst that started my course of change. At that time, if there was going to be any chance of stopping the abuse and saving our marriage and giving the children the family life they deserved, I needed to break my silence about the abuse that was being inflicted on me and the effect it was having on my behaviour. Silence had been my chief predator and was trying to kill me, just as Lucia Osborne-Crowley had experienced. Realising for the first time that keeping silent was literally killing me, it was time to change my thinking and start to speak up. They were harrowing memories.

Women who have killed themselves to stop the pain of abuse and the feelings of hopelessness have taken their stories with them. Sometimes they even take their children as well, feeling that there is no hope in this world for them either—so sad and tragic! I know that I didn't want to die; I just didn't want to live with the pain. I'm pleased that the pain didn't win that day and I'm still here for my family and for myself. I'm pleased that I have since furthered my need to break the silence and had the courage to make a statement to the police. By writing this book I have been able to tell my story, my trek, that may help other women to choose to live with new hope and meaning.

...grow

...toe to toe

...land

...embryo

...go

...understand

6

Resolving the Feelings of Shame

"Guilt is internally constructed, based on our knowledge of our-selves and the recognition that our behaviour has deviated from that self; shame, on the other hand, is given to us by others. Shame is inorganic. Guilt says, I made a mistake.
Shame says, I am a mistake."
—Lucia Osborne-Crowley, *I Choose Elena.*

ON RETURN FROM OUR holiday at the Gold Coast we thought we were ready to sort out all our problems, so Brian and I approached our Pastor and his wife. Our Pastor, shocked to hear what I had been enduring, challenged Brian to meet with him to find a solution to his dysfunctional sexual behaviour while I met with his wife to work through healing for my sustained trauma.

She suggested I go to a doctor to receive some medical support. This was a positive move because the doctor prescribed antidepressants for me. Over the following few months, this medication gradually enabled me to alter my outlook on how I was being treated and shift from what I can now call being in a "frozen" state to one of "flight." This transformed reaction empowered me to have the courage to say "no" to Brian's abusive sexual advances and, as a result, I did not have to endure his abuse anymore. As the medication started to take effect, the pastor's wife also suggested that, for my protection, Brian was not to touch me or make any sexual advances to me. This was hard for Brian to accept as, for him, a marriage was a license to have sexual contact. He was very reluctant to accept, but he finally did. Our respective families were told that we were experiencing relationship issues and were endeavouring to resolve them for an optimistic outcome.

The following Christmas, a family member visited us. In private she told me that Brian had sexually abused her on multiple occasions from when she was young until she was sixteen. I was horrified. The stories she shared involved him cornering her naked in a bathroom and touching her and ridiculing her body. He tried to have sexual intercourse with her, but she managed to fend him off. During this period of abuse, she tried to tell the adults what was going on but was never believed.

When I asked why she hadn't informed me before I was married, she explained that she believed he had changed. But after we shared our stories, it was clear to both of us that he had not changed in his sexual desires. It was obvious he did not value an intimate loving relationship with a wife and saw marriage merely as an opportunity to finally get his desires met. He had only locked his distorted thoughts away until, in his own mind, he had a marriage contract that gave him permission, even if it meant by force, to have what he had long desired: SEX!

Both my mother-and father-in-law continued to deny my allegations of their son's behaviour toward me. They never wavered in their total disbelief that their quiet, meek son could, in any way, behave in the manner I revealed. According to them, my accusations had to be fabrications to discredit his character so that I could get at his money. His family deserted me. This left me with only my family, who couldn't get their heads around the magnitude of the situation although they did try to support me. It was all too hard for people to cope with. No one seemed to want to know. So, the best way for everyone was to just ignore it and hope that we would sort out our relationship problems by ourselves and their need for involvement would go away. The whole time this was going on, I was struggling to look after four confused, suffering, secondary-school-aged children. I was doing this largely by myself, as Brian had withdrawn from his role as a father, using his usual passive-aggressive behaviour, and was totally unco-operative with me.

My sessions continued with the pastor's wife, while Brian was supposed to meet up with our pastor. But he only met him once. On one occasion though, when Brian met with one of the pastors at the church, I received a phone call. This pastor suggested that I come down and have a chat about how I wanted to be "loved" by Brian. *What a great opportunity for progress*, I thought. So I went down to the church, only to be met by these two men joking and making fun of me.

The pastor started with, "So, tell us how you want to be loved. Brian doesn't know, so how about you let him know."

I remember trying to say things like, "Helping me with the children and the housework," and, "Listening to me when I'm hurting. Respecting, and honouring me as a woman and responding in a helpful positive way."

The pastor's response was that Brian said he was already trying to do this but that I pushed him away and yelled and screamed at him *all* the time. They even laughed at me! I couldn't believe the mockery I was receiving from these men, especially considering one was a pastor who should have been in a position of care and empathy.

Where was equality with gender and compassion in this counselling to repair a fracturing family?

Breaking down, I blurted, "Well, how do you love your wife? Did you violently rape her on your wedding night? Do you sexually abuse her in her sleep? And emotionally and verbally abuse her if you don't get your way? Do you punish her with passive-aggressive behaviour instead of replying civilly to the first request at communicating? Do you bait her to have to repeat the request and increase the volume of her voice because she thinks you haven't heard her the first, second, third, or fourth time? Do you now brand her as a mad woman yelling and screaming? Do you leave all the domestic work for her to do, or do you ask how you can help? Do you get up early every Saturday and drive four children to four different sporting activities and then do the rounds to pick them all up again—or do you just leave it for her to do every week and every day? Do I need to go on? There is so much more I could say!"

By the end of this, the pastor was down on his knees in front of me, profusely apologising for his ignorance and naïvety. I was an emotional and physical wreck. Leaving them to discuss my explosive revelation, I hoped for some constructive outcome, but I never heard anything more from that pastor. Nor anything constructive from the head pastor. My plight was obviously too hard, and too complex, for them to handle!

Brian became more and more silent toward me. It was like walking on eggshells at home. Endeavouring to maintain my vow, I tried to do everything I could to make the marriage work and uphold the commitment I had made to stay with him for the whole of my life. The children, I felt, were better off living with both their parents together, but I knew they were suffering. I hated divorce due to the Biblical teaching that it was wrong for people to marry then walk away when the going got tough as the union of marriage was for life. The financial and emotional mess that resulted from split families tormented me. So I avoided any thought of that route, but I knew I wasn't coping with this stand-off and the shame associated with a failing marriage.

Brian had been saying for years that he may as well leave me if I wasn't going to give him the sex he wanted, to which I would reply, "Please don't talk like that, we can make it work."

Being on antidepressants enabled me to alter my outlook, and instead, I began to reply, "Well go then if you want to, I'm not stopping you."

I vividly remember his spontaneous response, "I'm not going anywhere."

With this complete turnaround in my reaction, I began to be able to contemplate and comprehend the implications. The antidepressants, I realised, were doing me some good. I even started saying to him, "Get yourself sorted out or you may as well get out. There are professionals who can help you but you have to decide that you want to get better."

Even after all this, I don't think he did much at all to help himself; he just continually blamed me for our problems.

I started becoming very fearful of his behaviour as he was so inward looking—first by disengaging, and then, out of the blue, he would have violent outbursts. I kept having nightmares of him killing me by smothering me with a pillow, which was not good for a well-rested sleep!

That Easter, his sister invited us to join her family and other friends at Ulladulla. We decided it would be good for the children to be around their cousins and for us to get away, but it was a long drive, and the children didn't travel well. At one point when I was driving, Jared and Nathan were having a fight in the back seat. Brian, sitting in the passenger seat, put his arm back to discipline Nathan and the boys fell very quiet. It wasn't until we stopped for lunch about an hour later that the awful damage Brian had inflicted on Nathan became evident to me. The index finger on his left hand had gone black and was swollen to over double its normal size. Brian had twisted Nathan's finger around and done immense damage.

Nathan wouldn't let me take him to a doctor once arriving at Ulladulla because, as he said, "He didn't want any ramifications to happen to his father." He suffered much pain and an inability to enjoy many of the activities during that holiday. His finger slowly healed over the next few months, but I don't think it has ever fully recovered.

The catalyst that finally made it inevitable that I needed to leave and separate was Brian challenging Nathan about changing the channel on the TV. Brian, seeing that a few of the children were watching the family room TV, went into the rumpus room where Nathan was watching a different show. Brian walked in and changed the channel; in response, Nathan pushed him away and changed the channel back. Brian grabbed Nathan and pushed him forcefully into the wall, breaking the plaster and creating a big hole. The shame I felt was palpable. Not only was I suffering terrible depression and fearing for my life, but now my children were also in danger. After my experience at the Gold Coast of wanting to jump out the window, the thought of suicide as a way out of my trauma was always there in my mind. The two options staring me in the face were that he would kill me, or I would kill myself, neither of which were favourable outcomes for the welfare of my children.

I had stopped caring much about myself at this point. Brian had done nothing to repair the damage he had caused our failing marriage and I had finally given up hope that it could be saved. The feelings of shame were saying to me that I was a mistake, just like my grandmother had told me. I had to let go of my marriage vow and my personal vow to disprove my grandmother, and admit I couldn't do it anymore, that I had failed, and that she was right. I had thought that sacrificing the last eighteen years of my life to keep my family together was the right decision to make, but it was evident that it was just too dangerous to continue. On admitting that I had to give up on my marriage, shame overwhelmed me. Shame had become my character.

Lucia Osborne Crowley writes in *I Choose Elena*:

> Guilt requires us to recognise that we have acted in a way that we regret, in a way that is out of character. This process is impossible for those who live with shame: for us, shame is our character. There is no sense in which we can act in a manner that is 'unlike ourselves' when we have no 'self' to speak of. Shame devours us from the inside out and leaves us empty: with no solid form, no edges, no boundaries, no structure. *(Osborne-Crowley 2020, 74).*

Emptiness did engulf me with no structure and no direction about how to move forward. I no longer knew who I was. All my decisions were for the sake of the children who were then sixteen, fifteen, and twelve. Brian and I had a meeting with our pastor's wife to talk through separation, during which it was agreed that it was to be a mutual decision to separate and not a case of me "kicking him out."

It seems that only I remember this meeting, as later Brian would say I told him to leave, and the pastor's wife conveniently couldn't remember. It is so sad when those who are supposed to be supporting you through a crisis don't even remember the details. It comes back to me, again and again, as being all my fault! To try and help me move forward, she said I needed to work through not judging Brian or his family, and to forgive him for what he had done to me. Forgiveness is a choice, and I had already chosen to forgive because I wanted to move forward and not be held back.

When contemplating where I would make a home for my children, I realised that moving was my only choice, so I bought land and commenced plans to build a new home. My parents were very supportive; they loaned me the deposit for the land and became guarantors for me to be able to secure a bank loan in my own right. Our home was put on the market with the hope that it wouldn't sell for a couple of months. It sold in ten days, however, and the purchaser wanted a two-month settlement! But the children and I needed somewhere to live before the new house was built, so Brian said he would take the children and I could "live in the gutter." This attitude of his—the lack of respect, putting me down, and controlling me—continued after our separation. Total destruction of the relationship ensued, and he would use the children in whichever way he could to degrade me and make me suffer.

I did not accept the original offer, so the purchaser came back with another offer, and I ended up signing a seven-month settlement at a lower price. My father paid Brian half the difference to encourage him to sign. My aim was for the least disruption of the children as possible with just one move, as Nathan was doing his VCE and Merryn was in Year Eleven by the time the seven months was up. Not good timing to move, but I felt I had no choice.

Church friends assisted us in moving to our new home and I cleaned our old house from top to bottom by myself, but the garage still needed to be attended to. Weeks before settlement, I asked Brian to come and clean out the garage as I had taken everything that I needed and left his stuff for him. As I had the keys, a time was made to meet him at the house to discuss the removal of the rest of his belongings from the garage. I didn't want to be on my own with Brian, so I asked my father to come for support. The three of us spent time looking at what was left, including some items of furniture and timber, but also quite a lot of rubbish that Brian had accumulated over the years. My father then said he would leave; I tried to tell him to stay so I wasn't alone with Brian, but he didn't understand my subtle messaging. After he left, Brian, who had been on his best behaviour while my father was there, became nasty and verbally aggressive.

Not feeling safe, I told him to please sort out his stuff in the garage, and that I would leave the garage door unlocked for him to access it. Then I left, assuming he would clean out the garage and leave the house ready for settlement.

The day before settlement was the same day as Merryn's Debutante Ball practice and I had to drive her to her girlfriend's place, as the mums were sharing the driving and I was picking them up afterwards. The Real Estate Agent called me late that afternoon to say that the purchaser had inspected the property, only to find the garage still full of stuff, and that the settlement would not go through if the garage contents weren't removed. Telling them that the contents were my ex-husband's, and that he was supposed to have removed it all, didn't make any difference. They just said they didn't care who removed it, it just needed to be done or the settlement would be defaulted. Panicking, I quickly called Brian and asked him to sort it. He said that he had removed all that he wanted to take, and the rest was my responsibility, then he hung up. I was furious and overwhelmed. What a typical action for him to try to derail the settlement and leave the mess for me to solve, knowing it would cause me stress and anxiety. I knew from his usual behaviour that I had to sort it out.

Knowing I didn't have much time, as I needed to take Merryn to her girlfriend's place, all I could think to do was ask the man who mowed my lawn to take everything to the tip for me. Understanding the urgency, he was so helpful and came straight away. Together, we quickly loaded his trailer and truck with the mess Brian had left. Some of it, including a bench, was quite heavy. Leaving him to complete the mammoth task, I rushed home to collect Merryn who was furious with me for making her late for her practice and holding up her friend and her mum. She had no interest in my explanation of the situation and wouldn't listen. As far as she was concerned, everything was my fault, and I should have better organised the clean up. Why does it inevitably seem to be the mother who always gets the blame? I had tried so hard to prepare Merryn for her Deb and make it an enjoyable memory for her, but it was being scarred by this disaster. The evening of the Deb was a few days later, and I endured the occasion, having to be around her spiteful father and family instead of relishing and enjoying my only daughter's milestone moment. She didn't want to be around me. I was heartbroken.

After a few months of counselling with our pastor's wife, she suggested I spend time with a trainee counsellor, and I spent many years after the split having sessions with her to help me through my many struggles, including looking after four teenagers on my own. The feelings of shame never left me. The shame of being divorced. The shame of yelling at my children to get them to do jobs around the house. The shame of not being the perfect mother I had vowed I would be. The shame of failure. The shame of being a mistake. Walking away from it all looked inviting at times, so I wouldn't have to have any contact with their father, but I had brought these children into the world and I was committed to them and to my responsibility to look after them and give them the best possible start in life, even in my circumstances. Their father wasn't capable of looking after them properly and I was simply being realistic about their welfare. He hadn't helped much when we were together, so there was no way he could look after these teenagers on his own. Staying alive for them was my only option.

Osborne-Crowley further writes in *I Choose Elena*:

> Once you experience this fight, flight, freeze response, particularly in a truly life-threatening situation, it lives on in your body and resurfaces again and again in everyday life. *(Osborne-Crowley, 2020, 75).*

That is exactly what happened to me. Every day was a struggle to get through. Brian continued his total destruction of any potential of us having a reasonable relationship for the sake of the children. He would use the children in whichever way he could in order to degrade me and make me suffer.

He tried not to pay me child support. He did lose his job through downsizing, then purposely phoned me to tell me that he wasn't going to get another job so that he didn't have to pay me any money. I experienced what poverty is like. If it wasn't for my parents helping to pay my mortgage, I would have lost the house.

In 2004, Nathan travelled overseas after completing university, Merryn was doing a different course as a gap year during her nursing degree, and the twins were studying their Year Twelve, when Brian rang me to tell me he was engaged to get married. It was very upsetting to hear that he was moving on in his life. To make the situation worse, he had not been paying child support for several years, nor was he having to cope with the constant care of the needs of the children—he was free to go courting while shirking his financial responsibilities!

While talking to my counsellor one day after church, Brian walked in hand-in-hand with his fiancée. Our pastor's wife immediately went over to congratulate them. I said to my counsellor, "How can she do that knowing all the awful treatment he has handed out to me?"

My counsellor's response was, "He is forgiven. If you can't forgive him and move on, you are the one with the problem."

I couldn't believe what I was hearing. My response to her was, "I thought you had to admit to your wrong doings, say sorry, ask for forgiveness, and then put it right by changing your actions with the person you have wronged. He has done none of these with me. Forgiving someone is a choice but it is a two-way street. The person you are forgiving has to make an effort to repair the damage."

Her response completely gutted me. Here was a man who had treated me appallingly, and now I was being told I was the one with the problem. Surely the pastor's wife was out of line by congratulating him without putting any pressure on him at all to make some effort in apologising to me and trying to repair our broken relationship? I was already having great doubts about this church and its teaching that God was against divorce and that forgiveness was always the answer. This incident just confirmed to me that it was this church and these teachings that were the problem, not me.

Our pastor and his wife had not put in any effort to make our split at least civil and manageable. Their solution, and other counsellors', was just to forgive, forget, and move on. But it wasn't working for me. My depression was getting worse and my ability to function properly and go to work was under extreme duress. Adding to my low self-esteem, I was suffering constant, severe headaches ever since I had moved to my new home. A specialist physician had put me in hospital on a cocktail of drugs. The numerous side effects of those drugs seemed only to add to my debilitating health issues.

My body was a mess. My relationship with my children was a mess. My plan was to get the twins through Year Twelve, then I was done. Forgiveness wasn't cutting it and shame had taken complete possession of me. Nathan returned from overseas and decided to go and live with his father, and soon after that the twins finished secondary school. Merryn came back from her course and continued her last year of her nursing degree. So, what did "I was done" look like? I had no idea!

It was at this time that I contacted the friend whom I had confided in many years before about the treatment I was experiencing from Brian. She had returned from living overseas for several years with her husband's work, so we caught up and reconnected. She told me that while living overseas, she had become a Catholic. Her story resonated with my feelings of frustration with the church I was attending, the questions that I was grappling with, and the lack of successful support I was receiving. The depth of this journey at this time of my life is too much for this book—as it is a book in itself—so I will leave the details for another time. Suffice to say, I had a new direction in my life just at the right time with my children being more independent and starting to leave the nest.

Still suffering from headaches, in desperation I visited a special naturopath. She picked up geopathic stress on my body and asked where my metre box was in my house. My answer was that it was on my bedroom wall right above the head of my bed. She said a metre box should never be on a bedroom wall, where you can spend more than eight hours every day. Thinking if that was bad, I asked her about the electricity substation that was situated next door and only a few metres away from my bedroom wall. Her eyes went to the ceiling and she exclaimed that I had to sell my house and move. In her opinion, that was the only way to improve my headaches and health. After living six-and-a-half years in that house, I finally did sell and move away, but I have suffered health issues ever since, mainly sensitivity to electromagnetic fields, including Wifi and powerlines. I still suffer from headaches, even though they aren't as frequent or as severe.

Just prior to selling the house, I had a big fight with Merryn over money. She couldn't obtain work after returning from her course and only had her Austudy and money from her father as income. She claimed she didn't have enough to give me any money towards board, but I couldn't afford to keep her.

Suffering from debilitating headaches and looking after the twins, I could only manage to work part time, so I just didn't have enough income to support everyone. That was all too much for her so she also went to live with her father and his wife. Only the twins moved with me to a rental property.

Nathan became engaged in 2007 and he asked me to give a speech at their engagement party, which I was thrilled to do. It was received positively, even quite emotionally, by them, other family members, and particularly by mothers of Nathan's friends from school whom he had become close to over the years. They said that I had spoken with great passion and love from the aspect of a mother's heart to her precious son and future daughter-in-law. On the following Monday though, I received a letter in the mail from Brian. He wrote:

The years of my marriage with you were filled with your persistent nagging, whining, yelling, and screaming, all of which I see now as an inappropriate way to behave. The way you treated me, and still continue to treat the children, is nothing short of emotional abuse.

The children have each, on their own, shared their pain and disappointment in the way you have behaved toward them and towards me. Someone you know well has shared that the way you treated me was very ugly. The things you have told the children have hurt and damaged them beyond belief, and you continue to do it. Emotional abuse is insidious and I suffered under it for many years. Then there was the issue of extreme sexual deprivation, which you used as another means of control and abuse. (I now have a normal and satisfying sex life!)

...Deirdre you really need to stop this continual rehashing of the past, flogging your side of the story. It is ugly and it is counterproductive for developing a friendly attitude towards each other for the sake of the children. I found your speech on Saturday night so hypocritical. You attempted to sell yourself as a "loving mother" but you are emotionally abusing your children with incessant yelling and nagging. Your behaviour has not been as perfect as you try to tell people.

He stated at the end of the letter that he had waited until after the engagement party to send this so anticipating my reaction did not spoil the kids' weekend.

When I received that letter, I cried and cried on the phone to my mother for over three hours, while she tried so desperately to keep me together and calm me down. The feeling of shame besieged me. I wanted to disappear and die. I felt so demoralised and worthless and swallowed every word he had used to describe me, even though I knew that he had twisted the truth.

What had I become and what did my children and others really think of me?

I had hoped that by separating I could get away from his clutches, but we had four children together and family gatherings were continually going to happen to celebrate special milestones. He still had power and control over me.

In Osborne-Crowley's second book, *My Body Keeps Your Secrets,* she writes:

> Holding on to shame means wearing the scars of a life spent fighting to be seen and understood and recognised and believed. It is constantly battling against voices telling you that you are not valid or honest or real. The thing about shame is that it eats at you until it fully consumes you. It's not just that you internalise the shame; rather, it becomes you. Shame is born out of the idea that there is a particular order to the universe that we must accede to if we are to live. It tells us there is a group armed with accepted wisdom that has the power to exclude us. Shame is a truly deadly emotion. It is pure evil. It is a liar.
>
> It is the emotion that supports and breathes life into every form of structural oppression we have ever created. It is the way that systematic unfairness gets under our skin and into our blood and bones. It is so powerful that we are never taught to question its authority. *(Osborne-Crowley 2021, 68-69)*

From my perspective, Osborne-Crowley describes shame exceedingly well. Her words were a revelation; they felt so true. My scar of shame had been continuously made deeper and consumed me for years. It kept my mouth shut—it success-fully silenced me! Shame created a prison for my being and immobilised my existence. It *was* my character.

To start a new life where no-one knew my perceived scarred and worthless background, I decided to try some study to expand my knowledge of the Catholic faith. This ultimately ended up being six years of part-time study which resulted in achieving a Bachelor of Theology, an achievement of which I'm extremely proud. Back in secondary school, I was told to not attempt HSC (now Year Twelve VCE) as I wouldn't pass due to my dyslexia and learning disabilities. It was during my second year in 2008 that I first met Ted. A relationship blossomed between us during 2009 and we were married in January 2010.

Ted has endured my highs and lows of behaviour and, at times, misinterpreted my needs for understanding, but even after some heartache we have managed to talk issues through and come out the other side, and he has stuck by me. It was Ted who saw me struggle with my granddaughters and told me that I shouldn't beat myself up if I couldn't look after them. It was he who witnessed the agony of my heart when I pushed myself to prove that I wasn't a failure when Merryn asked me to help with the girls. It was he who witnessed my anxiety when the children and Brian wanted Christmas together and who heard my statement that I wouldn't be coming if that happened.

It was he who came with me to counselling to work through my anguish of being around the man who wanted to play happy families for Christmas—this same man who had raped me, his twenty-one-year-old bride, on their wedding night—because I didn't want to spend Christmas with my abuser. It was he who witnessed the nasty letters and texts from Brian to try and control me. It was he who witnessed Brian and his wife always stating, "for the sake of the children," do everything "for the sake of the children." It was he who witnessed Brian's speech at Rohan's wedding that showed him just how much of a narcissist Brian is. It was he who witnessed Brian's wife insisting at Jared's wedding that she sit in the seat reserved for the mother of the groom. It was he who witnessed the way Brian and his wife used the children to upset their mother. It was he who watched me struggle just being around Brian at family birthdays. It was he who saw the effects of the news items that kept coming of the stories of women who had been sexually manipulated by Harvey Weinstein. It was he who watched me cry in front of the TV as the onslaught ensued of more stories from women with the *#MeToo* movement. It was he who suggested I could have PTSD, and insisted I go to the doctor and get a diagnosis. It was he who has come with me to many of my counselling sessions to help manage my ailing mental health. It was he who supported me to make the decision to go to the police and make a statement. It was he who said it was about time we change the rhetoric from "for the sake of the children" to, "for the sake of Deirdre." It is Ted who has supported me to stay alive by loving me and suggesting that we move to the beach for the improvement of my wellbeing.

Words can't express the difference of journeying through this struggle when someone is standing by you. It is hard to continually exist, but more bearable doing it with someone who sympathises with you and who talks through the many issues with you. My heart goes out to all those women existing on their own or with children. I did it for ten years on my own while trying to manage the children, and I know what agony it is. Even saying you are "surviving" is not the right word. I hate using that word. I was not surviving; I was only existing. I'm so grateful for Ted's ongoing support.

In preparation to explain to my children why I had gone to the police, I wrote a letter in consultation with my counsellor from ECASA. I wanted them to understand that I wasn't doing it out of a desire for revenge, money, or compensation but purely to be able to recover my mental health. As I had become more aware of the depth of the damage on my mental health from the abuse triggered by their father, causing me to be unable to work and function normally in my daily life, it was the right time to speak up and break the silence that was destroying me. It was right *for me* to be part of the voice of women, to tell our stories, to be believed and make a difference for societal change. It is time that perpetrators should be made accountable for their behaviour and for women to deserve justice. I hoped that by going to the police, Brian would admit to the damage he had caused me, that I would receive a lasting authentic apology, to which I would say that I forgive him—as I already have done—and that he would endeavour to have an ongoing civil relationship with me where he would treat me with respect and dignity "for the sake of the children" *and* "for the sake of Deirdre." If he had miraculously changed his leopard spots and admitted to his behaviour, given me a lasting authentic apology, asked for forgiveness, and showed that he was going to treat me with respect and dignity, then I would have withdrawn my complaint to the police and gone on to enjoy a renewed lasting relationship with him and the children!

My counsellor continued to support me during the months of waiting for the police to interview Brian, the pastor and his wife, the girlfriend who had been the only one I had told during the abuse, another friend, and the children. She said I needed to be able to recall the abuse if my case were to go to court. This was a daunting prospect that I was not looking forward to but was prepared to do if it came to that.

After eighteen months of waiting for the police to get back to me, I received a phone call for me to come in and meet with the Senior Constable. My hopes were high for progress after waiting so long and enduring the fallout. Ted accompanied me for support. The Senior Constable was holding a massive file for my case, which looked impressive, but my anticipation was quickly dashed when he announced that his superior had made the decision not to proceed with my case due to insufficient evidence. It took both of us a moment to realise what he was saying, and I was suddenly overwhelmed with despair. I broke down, crying hysterically, unable to be pacified, and the Senior Constable asked Ted if he should call a counsellor to try and calm me down. The Senior Constable quickly briefed her on the situation and my condition before she entered the room. She was the loveliest person to speak to at that gut-wrenching time. After about an hour, she had put some equilibrium back into my being and reassured me that I had done the right thing by reporting my case to the police, and that I was believed. Speaking with the Senior Constable again, I was able to get a better understanding of the proceedings. He said that at Brian's first interview he answered everything as "No comment," meaning that the case would then have automatically gone to trial once they had interviewed all the other witnesses.

Then, a few months later, Brian asked for a second interview, which he was granted. At this interview he did answer the questions. The only admission he made was the rape on the wedding night in Launceston. However, I knew that under the Crimes Act in Tasmania in 1981, it was not a crime to rape your wife. I feel incredulous to live in a country that still had such archaic laws around the treatment of women back in the 1980s. What is the difference between raping your girlfriend one night and being found guilty of a crime, but raping your wife the next night and it not being considered a crime—simply because you are now married? It's incomprehensible.

Regarding the other alleged rapes that occurred in my sleep, Brian stated that was how we "did it" as a couple, so he had believed that I was consenting as his wife. His denial of any other abuse or assaults toward me meant they believed that they had no worthwhile admission from him to take to a judge. It was a crime, by then, to rape your wife in Victoria, but the police didn't feel that they had enough evidence to succeed at a trial, even though they felt he was guilty and some of the witnesses who had heard him admitting to his conduct either could not, or chose not to, remember! The leopard has not changed its spots.

I continued to struggle with feeling I had been let down by the police and, more so, by the witnesses who could have assisted me with the truth. If forgiveness was all that I needed to do, why was I still in so much pain with shame enveloping me? And why was I still struggling with the relationships of the people who I love so much and wanted to be loved by? Just as Osborne-Crowley states in her book about shame, I felt that the systematic unfairness had got under my skin into my blood and bones and was consuming me. I had no right to justice as I was unworthy. I couldn't talk to anyone at this time except Ted, my counsellor, and my cousin.

...wise

...pain

...price

...gained

...anything

7

Overcoming the Effects of Post Traumatic Stress Disorder

*"Trauma sufferers tend to identify themselves as survivors,
rather than as animals with an instinctual power to heal."*
—Peter A. Levine, *Waking The Tiger: Healing Trauma*

As human beings, we are privileged to have been gifted with
the most advanced brain in the animal kingdom, but the mores
of society have, unfortunately, caused our species to ignore
our instinctive animal abilities most of the time. Our societal
custom has been to just get on with life by being superhuman,
through portraying a stiff upper lip of confidence while ignor-
ing the source of debilitating symptoms caused by traumatic

experiences. This culture has stopped us from recognising that we have the instinctual ability to end the symptomatic effect of trauma. It has caused our bodies to become ill, our behaviour to go awry, and the loss of ability to reach our human gifted potential.

Peter Levine, who holds a Ph.D. in Medical and Biological Physics from the University of California at Berkeley and is an expert in psychology, stress, trauma, and pain management, describes the three parts of the human brain in his book *Waking the Tiger: Healing Trauma*:

> The involuntary and instinctual portions of the human brain and nervous system are virtually identical to those of other mammals and even reptiles. Our brain, often called the triune brain, consists of three integral systems. The three parts are commonly known as the reptilian brain (instinctual), the mammalian or limbic brain (emotional), and the human brain or neo-cortex (rational). *(Levine 1997, 17)*

Pre-historic human beings were hunters but were also aware of being hunted, and this has caused the dilemma of when to fight or when to flee. Human beings don't have the agility of an impala, or the sleek physic of a fast-running cheetah with its matching fangs and claws to enhance its predator abilities. However, once humankind began gathering in tribal groups, inventing tools for trades, weapons for defence and hunting, and utilising the benefits of fire and pooled resources, our chances of surviving were enormously enhanced. But the confusion in our brains to process life-threatening situations still remained.

When we are challenged with a life-threatening event, our rational brains may become blurred, resulting in our instinctual brain causing us to become immobile or retreat to a frozen state. Being in a frozen state can cause pent-up energy to be trapped in the nervous system that can wreak havoc in our bodies and may cause our brains to struggle and, thus, make irrational decisions.

The Autonomic Nervous System (ANS) can be continually aroused even when the threat has long gone, but to the victim it feels like the traumatic event is happening over and over again in the present. The energy locked in the ANS manifests in the emotions of fear and anxiety, and becomes a vicious cycle that repeats itself and causes immobility that prevents the completion of the natural resolution, even though the initial threat is over. The memory can go awry. Explicit memories, ones that are readily recalled and require words to describe events, can keep a traumatic event always in the front of a person's mind to be replayed often. These events may include facts that are said either aloud or in the mind, or written down. Whereas implicit memories, ones that are not conscious and have to do with recalling repeated procedures that we use in everyday life without having to think about it—like riding a bike or tying our shoelaces—will be recalled by a healthy individual without any discomfort. But to an individual who has suffered a trauma, recalling implicit memories can be confusing and involve unnerving bodily sensations and disconcerting emotions. The traumatic memories can be stored in the brain and evoked as somatic (from the Greek word *soma* which means "the living body") memories, ones that show sensations in the body instead of the mind. The body remembers but not the mind. These implicit memories can be recalled by the trigger of a song, taste, smell, touch, sound, movement, colour, or sight and, in normal circumstances, would be an enjoyable positive experience. But in the case of a recalled trauma, the recall can be a harrowing negative encounter without the person understanding where it has come from.

The *Diagnostic and Statistical Manual of Mental Disorders 5th edition* (DSM-5) describes someone who has experienced a traumatic event, causing them to manifest these psychological negative memory symptoms, as a person suffering from Post Traumatic Stress Disorder (PTSD). This anxiety disorder develops in response to an event that has exposed the person to "actual or threatened death, serious injury, or sexual violence...directly experiencing the traumatic event(s)." (*American Psychiatric Association 2022, 271-275*).

They experience intrusive symptoms that cause distressing memories of the traumatic event, and so they try to avoid external reminders that may arouse these distressing memories. A formal diagnosis of PTSD can be made when there are significant symptoms resulting in the declining of a person's social and/or occupational ability to function normally for at least one month. This can happen as early as six months after the traumatic event or can become apparent many years later, which may happen after a trigger has awakened the memories of the event.

Typically, symptoms of PTSD sufferers include: sleep disturbances; mood swings; being quick tempered (usually expressed through yelling, getting into fights or damaging objects); flashbacks; avoidance of certain activities; becoming socially withdrawn; having suicidal thoughts; amnesia (especially about the traumatic event); fatigue; inability to concentrate; inability to feel pleasure; depression that can include a lack of having positive emotions; a substantial increase in negative emotions such as fear, guilt, shame and confusion; anxiety; detachment and estrangement from other people; and hyper-arousal in response to trauma related stimuli that can increase the person's blood pressure or heart rate, as well as causing hyperventilating.

These symptoms cannot be attributed to a head injury, or some other explained medical condition, or medication, or non-prescription drug taking or abuse of alcohol. These last two can become a means to try and escape from negative symptoms but then they are not the initial cause.

A normal person's activation of their ANS response to the initiation of a stressful event will be to manage the rise and fall of their stress level, as the stressful event happens and then passes. But in a PTSD sufferer, their Sympathetic Nervous System, that is part of their ANS, is already on high alert. So when more stress is activated on the PTSD sufferer, it is highly likely that they will be pushed past their coping level. This can cause them to suffer feelings of being overwhelmed or help-less, which can become long lasting or even permanent. These constant bouts of overwhelm may cause those diagnosed with PTSD to suffer from substance abuse by using illicit drugs or alcohol to try and suppress their levels of anxiety and their feelings of not being able to cope. This substance abuse just adds more issues to their compounding symptoms.

As the permanency of chronic helplessness becomes the norm, which means existing constantly in a frozen state, the sufferer is likely to keep following pre-determined dysfunc-tional behaviour. This becomes a vicious cycle of victimisa-tion without the sufferer fully understanding the reason why their dysfunctional behaviour and self-loathing even exists. Immobility can keep a sufferer in a relationship where they are dominated and, as a result, are repeatedly abused and suffer more trauma. Sufferers are often unable to break their habitual behaviour. They feel trapped and powerless to move through the frozen immobility response, resulting in their enduring more anxiety, shame, numbness, depression, and detachment from themselves.

Even what seems like trivial issues to one person can very quickly become huge problems to a sufferer, who may frequently experience panic and dread with just normal life circumstances. The mind might not consciously understand the effect of the trauma on a sufferer, but the body certainly does. This shows up in all sorts of ways, such as chronic illnesses, debilitating symptoms, and inappropriate behaviour. Much of the violence witnessed by our communities can be attributed, directly or indirectly, to unresolved traumas in people. These are people who are desperately trying, albeit unsuccessfully, to get their equilibrium back under control and re-establish empowerment in their lives. But they are unconsciously looking for answers in the wrong place, such as through revenge on society or external illicit influences, instead of finding the answers from within themselves.

To be able to commence transformation, a PTSD sufferer must first admit and acknowledge that they have suffered a traumatic event. This may be very harrowing for a sufferer who has been trying ever since the traumatic event to forget it ever happened, or may not even be aware that it did happen.

Nevertheless, they are suffering from its effects. Professional assistance is highly recommended to recall the dreadful memories of the encounter or encounters, to prevent them from being re-traumatised, and to work through the details of their experience. Once they have recalled their memories, they must own it as their experience and verbalise that they have been a victim.

It may take quite some time for a sufferer to work through to recall their memories and accept that the trauma happened to them and the memories are real. Many try for so long to not think of themselves as a victim, as they perceive that society doesn't like the "victim mentality." Yet this strategy just compounds the sufferer's agony. However, once a sufferer has worked through the stage of their acknowledgement and acceptance, they must not remain a "victim," otherwise the healing process gets stuck, and progress is not made. So many sufferers, especially sexual abuse sufferers, use the terminology that they are a sexual abuse "survivor" and are proud to be called that. They can lose the will or the impetus to move on to the next stage of healing. The media should also be challenged in their responsibility in changing societal perception and stopping the use of the word "survivor." Fuelling its continual usage may be affecting the healing and recovery progress of many people who have suffered sexual abuse.

Further to advancing from recalling memories of abuse and accepting the "victim stage," PTSD sufferers can try Cognitive Processing Therapy (CPT) with a professional trained in the therapy. This therapy can also help in recalling memories and assist with the sufferer's "stuck points" that may be holding them back from achieving healing. This experience can still be very harrowing and time consuming (it can take over twelve weeks), but it may be what a sufferer requires to be able to move forward. Unfortunately though, re-traumatising can occur, in which case the therapy would need to stop to prevent the sufferer being worse off.

Alternatively, we can endeavour to get back to our animal instinctual abilities to heal and progress past the victim/survivor stage. Levine puts it so well in his book, namely showing that animals are our teachers for our health and vigour. As he explains:

> One of the difficulties in treating trauma has been the undue focus on the content of an event that has engendered trauma. Trauma sufferers tend to identify themselves as survivors, rather than as animals with an instinctual power to heal. The animal's ability to rebound from threat can serve as a model for humans. It gives us a direction that may point the way to our own innate healing abilities.

We must pay attention to our animal nature to find the instinctive strategies needed to release us from trauma's debilitating effects. *(Levine 1997, 98)*

Levine is saying that for a PTSD sufferer to be able to achieve progress in healing, they should decide that they desire to be healed. This may sound silly, but it isn't. Many sufferers get used to their way of life and don't investigate for positive change. Also, people who are addicted to alcohol or drugs may find it hard to break this addiction without professional assistance. But the reward of a more fulfilling life and better relationships should be a strong drawcard.

The realisation that nature and our animal instinct hasn't been lost from our humanity, even though we have the tendency to forget it, will give the trauma sufferer power to draw upon this animal instinct for healing. The nervous system of trauma sufferers isn't damaged, rather it is frozen and immobilised, and the natural rhythm needs to be completed.

To encompass our innate ability to complete our immobilised nervous system after trauma, we can use our "felt sense," as first described by the American philosopher, Eugene Gendlin in his book *Focusing*, published in 1978.

Levine has utilised Gendlin's theory in his own development of trauma treatment and expresses the process thus:

As we begin the healing process, we use what is known as the "felt sense," or internal body sensations. These sensations serve as a portal through which we find the symptoms, or reflections, of trauma. In directing our attention to these internal body sensations, rather than attacking the trauma head-on, we can unbind and free the energies that have been held in check. *(Levine 1997, 66)*

Even if we aren't aware of it, we are constantly processing information from our environment with subtle nuances telling us where we are and how we feel about it. The felt sense combines these subtle nuances and other scattered information to give meaning to us about an experience. Levine uses the analogy of listening to music where we concentrate on the total aural experience and not on every single note. By using our physical senses of sight, sound, smell, touch, and taste, we are assisted in gathering the information that contributes to our felt sense. Internal perceptions of muscle tension or movement and body temperature also add data to our felt sense along with our thoughts. But rather than being a thought, it is a feeling or a sensation. Language finds it difficult to communicate just what felt sense is, as it is subtle, complex, ever-changing, and intricate.

Sometimes we say, "I felt it in my waters" to explain a sensation. This is because we struggle to describe the feeling in words. Much of the time we take the sensations in our body for granted and are unaware of them due to their subtleness and obscurity.

Think about the joy we feel when we're out in the bush, watching a waterfall tumble over a rocky ledge and crash below in a burst of spray and sound, before the water continues its journey down a bush-lined gully. We watch the spray as it creates a rainbow, adding vibrant colour and enjoyment to the scene. The gentle breeze moves through the eucalyptus and acacia trees lining the hills of the gully, giving off that strong, familiar Australian bush smell that permeates the air. A sense also notices the sounds of birds calling to each other, adding to the sounds heard over the crashing water. The air is fresh and fragrant and we breathe in big breaths of the refreshing smell. We feel the cool dampness of the spray of water that has landed on our skin. Time is spent sitting and soaking up the bodily sensations that are aroused by the atmosphere.

So many of our physical senses have been in play as we enjoy our surroundings, but our "felt sense" would also be working overtime. The awe and wonder of the experience would be relaxing our tight muscles from the stress of life, but we don't consciously think about it, we just enjoy the peace and tranquillity it gives our body and how relaxing the experience makes us feel.

How many times have we walked along a bush track or through parkland and felt that we are being followed? We turn around and no one is there. But a short time later someone catches up and passes us. How did we know that there was someone coming? I didn't think I heard anything but I must have sensed the presence of someone there. The Australian First Nations People knew how to use their felt sense when tracking prey and being cautious that they were not being hunted themselves. They certainly had skills for surviving in the harsh Australian country that the early European settlers had no idea about as they weren't adept in how to utilise their felt sense in this unfamiliar environment.

Kangaroos graze calmly, enjoying their docile existence. Then their felt sense picks up danger, and they become vigilant with their heads shooting up and their ears moving around as they try to pick up other information through sight and hearing to enhance their felt sense to ascertain whether there is the need to fight, flee, or freeze. The danger seems to pass and the kangaroos' bodies give a shudder and a twitching spasm before they get back to grazing. This is actively repeated many times during the day.

A short while later, the mob of kangaroos again sense danger, and again their heads shoot up, their ears move around, but this time the kangaroos sense the advancement of a pack of dingoes slowly stalking towards the mob. If the dingoes decide to move in and attack, the mob use their unconscious instinct through their reptilian and limbic brains as to whether they are going to remain stationary and fight back or decide to hop away and go into flight mode instead. Deciding to bound away, most of the kangaroos are fast enough to escape from the dingo pack, but one young, slower kangaroo is caught by the pack of dingoes. The kangaroo, realising it is futile to try and fight and knowing it's not about winning but surviving, goes into freeze mode.

Sometimes an animal that goes into the immobility stage does so to imitate they are dead. By doing this they are hoping that their attackers will give up the fight, thinking that they are already dead and that the meat may be bad so, with no advantage to continue the attack, they move away.

After some time, this enables the kangaroo the chance to escape and shake off the attack, by twitching and shuddering to release their body of the energy built up caused by the trauma of the near-death experience. The cycle is complete with no lasting traumatic effect being left with the kangaroo, who can then re-join the mob. If the dingoes do continue and kill the kangaroo, the immobility of the frozen state assists the muscles to be relaxed, which helps the kangaroo experience a less painful death.

As humans, we too have the same instinct of felt sense when we are threatened with a dangerous encounter. We must decide whether we have the power and resources to fight back, flee from the scene, or go into an immobile frozen state to endure the threat. If we have the strength or resources to fight back or be able to flee from the perceived threat of danger, and the energy required is released and not stored in the body, then no traumatic effect will be retained by the body in the nervous system. But if the threat of danger is perceived as real, and pre-conditioning stops us from reacting, or we just decide we can't fight or can't escape by fleeing, the body goes into a frozen immobile state. This means the energy that hasn't been able to be released will be stored in the nervous system and will cause symptoms of trauma in the body.

The difference between us and the animal instinct for responding to a traumatic threat is our predominant human neo-cortex rational brain. This would normally give us superior productive ability, but it can take control and interfere with the animal instinctual impulses of our reptilian and limbic parts of our brain. The emotions of fear and anxiety can bring about a constant cycle of immobility that impairs the instinctual cycle to be completed naturally. The body of the PTSD sufferer believes that it is still under threat, causing the effect of traumatic symptoms. By using the felt sense of the symptoms caused by the trauma as sensations in the body, a change of empowerment can start to release the pent-up energy that needs to be released and allow the completion of the instinctual cycle.

By drawing on these animal instincts within us—that may require help to complete the cycle that is trapped in the body—the PTSD sufferer can seek professional guidance to complete this process.

Utilising the work of Dr Peter Levine, Somatic Experiencing (SE) recognises the importance of the messages the body gives us, that other verbal therapies do not tap into. The body and the mind are so entwined that traumatic experiences frozen in the body can be released through somatic psychotherapy by using tools and techniques to tap into the physical sensations locked away in the body. Thus, it frees the sufferer from the incomplete state that has been stymied from running its course.

This empowerment can be either subtle and slow, or impactful in a sudden intense episode of trembling and shaking as the brain activates the awareness of felt-sense sensations. The progress of the mind and soul processing the energy that is being released from the nervous system is the sign that success is being achieved.

The journey of healing will not be immediate, just as the effect of the trauma has developed over time, especially if there have been repeated traumas, but any advancement is to be celebrated when success can be sighted. A fulfilling life of enjoyment and satisfaction is the reward of determination and persistence to find a way through the mire of a perpetual debilitating merry-go-round of symptoms of trauma.

Recognising the cause of symptoms in the body of the PTSD sufferer, and understanding our instinctual animal ability to break the perpetual cycle through our felt sense, are valuable insights. However, there are still many more factors to consider for the PTSD sufferer for healing to progress and for positive results to be achieved.

...strong

...invincible

...woman

8

Beginnings of a New Life

"The truth is that success is found in the tiniest increments, the smallest moments that build up to a new life."
—Lucia Osborne-Crowley *My Body Keeps Your Secrets*

Reading Osborne-Crowley's book taught me that silence is a deadly predator, and shame is its close brother. I had broken the silence but I had not found a way to deal with the shame that still possessed me. So, I decided that having experienced the revelation I received on Easter Sunday at low tide out on the rocks about the effects on me of the behaviour of my mother and grandmother and the implications with my sister, I would write down my revelation and send it as a letter to my parents. I wasn't sure how they would receive it. But I knew I had to write it, putting in as much detail as I felt was appropriate. My father rang Ted a few times to check on me, which I greatly appreciated, and said he was very pleased that I had had the courage to write the letter, albeit very sad for them to read, but they understood my need to open-up. He was prepared to wait for me to be ready to talk to him again on the phone. It took me about two weeks to call him and we had a good chat without discussing the letter. My wellbeing needed to improve before that was going to happen as I was too fragile, but progress was being made. We were talking again.

So, I was admitting to the hurt I had experienced from my earliest memories and from Brian's sexual abuse, and had stopped the silence, but I wasn't sure how to deal with the pain of shame. Trying to grasp more insight I re-read Osborne-Crowley's words:

> Guilt is internally constructed, based on our knowledge of ourselves and the recognition that our behaviour has deviated from that self; shame, on the other hand, is given to us by others. Shame is inorganic. Guilt says, I made a mistake. Shame says, I am a mistake. *(Osborne-Crowley 2021, 74).*

Reading and re-reading the words, "shame on the other hand is given to us by others." I had an inspired perception.

So I asked myself this question: *Is it possible to figuratively give shame that is weighing me down back to the other person, since, as it is their guilt, why should I be carrying the burden as my shame?* I thought about Brian who seemed to have no remorse at all about what he had done to me. Then, in my mind, I gave him my feelings of shame, and gave it back to him as his guilt of his behaviour toward me. Wow! That was liberating and so simple to do! I just had to believe it. I thought: *Why not try it with my grandmother as well?*

As a child, I holidayed with my family, not far away from where I now live at Balnarring Beach. My grandmother was always with us, and this was where most of her abuse took place. Walking around to the place where we holidayed, I sat on a log and, even though she has long gone physically from my life, I started to talk to her as if she was there again in person. Using my felt sense to connect with the vision of her being there, I realised I had the sensation of a knot in my stomach. Verbalising to her about what she had done to hurt me, the silence was being broken and I was admitting to my soul—and her—what effects I had experienced from her abuse. Figuratively, in my mind, I took my feelings of shame and gave them back to her as her guilt. I forgave her in my heart.

I asked her if she now admitted to her actions towards me and whether she was sorry for what she had done to me? Of course, she wasn't there to answer me, and I wasn't trying to communicate with the dead like in a séance. So, I answered for her. It didn't feel right to just leave guilt hanging on her and I felt that if she were here now, she would be sorry for what she had done to me and would ask to be forgiven as she would be enlightened by knowing the magnitude of the effect on my life. Just gazing there, looking at the property, I remembered so vividly my holidays there as a child, and reflected on my interaction with my grandmother and a few positive experiences with her.

Watching the wind in the trees, I pondered about our dead ancestors and whether they can hear us—not a particularly spiritual moment, more a curious thought. Our ancestors lived and they died. The lifetime of each generation overlaps with the one before and the one after. This was a location in which my grandmother had lived and walked, and I was connecting with my identity from my past. Nonetheless, I didn't need to be affected by it anymore; instead I only needed to see the positive.

Being immensely buoyed by the experience of communicating with my grandmother in this way, I felt that I could believe that the internal vow that I had made many years ago of proving I wasn't a failure and would make a success of my life, was finally lifted from me.

There was nothing to prove to her or anyone else anymore. Discerning that I am not a failure, nor a mistake—and

I never was and I never had to prove it—was incredibly liberating. I felt the relief in my body. Striving for perfection to justify my existence wasn't necessary anymore. Wow! I could feel I was making progress. My body became relaxed and my stomach knot disappeared. A feeling of peace came over me.

Understanding that forgiveness, as being an essential component in the process of healing, is paramount, but grasping that there are crucially more steps in the process, was exciting my soul for the potential of a positive freeing outcome. Deciding I needed to quickly write down these steps that were having a huge beneficial effect on healing my mental wellbeing and quality of life, I strode back home. This is what I wrote:

The steps to assist in dealing with an abusive past:

- Admit to the hurt that was caused to you, by whom, name the abuse, describe it and the effect it has had on you;

- Break the silence and tell someone you can trust, such as a counsellor, friend, family, or even the police;

- Figuratively give back to the abuser your feelings of shame that the hurt has caused, as it is their guilt and their responsibility;

- Forgive them for their actions. If the person has passed away, mediate for them and answer that they are sorry and have asked for forgiveness, or if they are still around but not involved in your progress, believe the guilt is back in their court.

If the abuser has been involved in the process, and also wants healing from their guilt, then their steps would be:

- Admit to the hurt they have caused, name the abuse, and describe it and the effect it has had on the victim;

- Apologise with a genuine and permanent apology;

- Ask for forgiveness of the victim who would then respond favourably;

- Change behaviour with positive actions towards the victim to make right on a continual basis without rehashing the past, otherwise that would then prove the apology is not genuine and permanent.

Better comprehending these steps, I contemplated them further with regard to the "Brian scenario." I knew I had already admitted to the hurt he had inflicted on me; I had broken the silence by talking to several counsellors, to some family and friends, and by going to the police; I had figuratively handed back to him my feelings of shame as it was his guilt that I didn't want anymore; I had already chosen to forgive him many times for his abusive behaviour towards me, but to renew it again was a good feeling. These steps seemed so simple, yet extremely effective for my wellbeing. I knew it was back in his court now, not mine. I could feel a weight being lifted from me, and I'm so much better so far, but I knew it was a process and could take time.

For a true and enduring reconciliation between parties, there needs to be a two-way dialogue. This has not happened to me yet, but I can always be hopeful that it will happen one day even though, from my experience, this leopard does not change its spots. What would need to happen is: admission of guilt by the guilty party, an apology, asking for forgiveness, and then actions to make it right. Without the action of changed behaviour then the apology is hollow and inauthentic.

To complete the reconciliation, the abused party would then need to say they accept the apology, offer forgiveness, and even make suggestions as to the action that could take place on an on-going basis. A guilty party reverting to their previous behaviour indicates that any apology was never authentic.

At this stage, while I was pondering all this, I remembered that Brian actually gave me a letter about two years after we separated in which he apologised to me for what he had done to me, and itemised different aspects of his abuse of me. That letter was his attempt to apologise but I have never seen it as being authentic because his behaviour straight after giving it to me, and since, has never shown that he ever meant what he wrote. So I feel that decisive action with a real change from abusive behaviour, both written and verbal sniping, to genuine positive interaction is what shows that a "sorry" is authentic.

In Brian's case, even though the sexual abuse had ceased, the emotional control continued. Therefore, the apology stage would need to be followed by constructive action and a change of behaviour that reflects a true change of attitude. I have been told many times by many people that all I needed to do was just forgive Brian, and then his hold over me would be released and I should be able to get on with my life. But this has proven to not work. I now know from experience that this process is flawed and incomplete. Brian not admitting to his abuse, giving no genuine apology, nor asking for forgiveness, and then making no change in his actions towards me, meant that I was stuck with his hold over me and unable to move forward. The perpetrator has had no problem getting on with his life, remarrying, and having a great time with our children. Whereas the poor victim is stuck with low self-esteem and suffering terribly from ailing mental health and physical ailments that affect many relationships.

But it was exciting to have found a lasting solution, an answer to this debilitating control and depression.

Exhilarating and liberating! Writing all this down has been so positive for me!

My next move was to follow up with my parents about my letter. It was a harrowing discussion to bring up the sad memories of my mother's behaviour and the effects that it had had on me. It was also harrowing for my mother, but was a liberating and healing time for all of us, where she apologised for hurting me and I forgave her. We were able to further discuss the effects on me from the abuse from my grandmother and I was enlightened as to how my mother had also been affected by her mother when she was a child, which had contributed immensely to her demeanour and behaviour. My letter opened in-depth discussion of issues we had never attempted to address before, and it produced an enormously positive outcome. The reward for me was life-changing and included a better relationship between myself and my parents. It also enabled topics never mentioned before to be raised with my sister about our grandmother. We were able to discuss my perception of our grandmother's favouritism toward my sister and she was able to state that she had been completely unaware that this had happened—another time of openness and healing of very important family relationships.

I felt that, little by little, I was finding some semblance of peace and contentment in my life, and success in finding answers for recovery. Osborne-Crowley wrote in her second book, *My Body Keeps Your Secrets,* that she realised that it was the small wins that helped with healing. She says:

I am struck by a thought I have had over and over and over again while writing this book. We are always taught that success looks like big moments and breakthroughs, big achievements, stages, applause, promotions, weddings, books. But it isn't. The truth is that success is found in the tiniest increments, the smallest moments that build up to a new life. *(Osborne-Crowley 2021, 290)*

I completely agree with her sentiments. I, too, was finding that the small increments of success and revelations were building up to a healthier wellbeing in my recovery.

I'm so relieved to have ultimately had that conversation with my parents when I did, especially with my mother, as her health did deteriorate quickly with dementia, and she would cognitively have been unable to successfully engage in that conversation. Sometimes the decision of having hard conversations with loved ones needs to be made before it is too late, otherwise the chance can be missed. I dearly love my mother and did physically lose her in September 2023. I have no regrets for having revealed to her my painful memories and feelings and having had the opportunity to forgive her while she was cognitively able to receive that forgiveness from me.

As for Brian, through discussion with my counsellor, it was decided that I would not go to any family functions where Brian and his wife would be present, to protect my mental health against his subjective taunts. This decision, even though it has proven difficult for the children to navigate, and meant I have missed out on those important grandchildren's birthdays, and school grandparent days, ultimately has been a positive choice to protect the progress of my healing and my new mantra, "For the sake of Deirdre." It has been up to the children how they choose to handle the situation of my stating that I won't be attending. I have, on occasions, had a separate catch up over a meal or received a video of them opening my present to them, which has been lovely. It has been my choice and my exercise of power—more small increments of progress to my new life.

Time passed, however, and the motivation to continue achieving progress with healing was urging me to explore further. I had researched Peter Levine's book *Waking the Tiger* and thought I understood his theory of using our senses as a human animal, but I had not experienced assistance with a trained therapist. Progress was happening but complacency can stall more small increments. I questioned whether it was time to try something different to be able to get back to family occasions, and so decided to explore finding a therapist that utilised Peter Levine's theories.

I found a therapist not far from home so I booked an appointment. Moniquea, a qualified Somatic Psychotherapist who specialised in Peter Levine's research, has been an immense support to unlock the "felt sense" and the sensations that portrayed what was trapped within me.

At first, when Moniquea invited me to notice what I felt in my body as I recalled the trauma of my wedding night, I could only say that I felt nothing. I had wanted there to be a dramatic sensation but I truthfully had to reply that there was no reaction. She explained that this was my nervous system's way of protecting me, an intelligent immobility that had helped me survive when I couldn't escape or fight. Together, we worked slowly and safely to bring awareness to small sensations such as a flutter in my chest, a subtle tightening in my throat, and a warmth in my arms.

Rather than reliving the event, Moniquea guided me to stay anchored in the present while sensing these impulses with curiosity. At times, as my body began to trust that it was safe, I could feel the stirring of the natural fight energy that had once been held back. With care and attunement, we explored this impulse through gentle, contained pushing motions with our hands, not as a re-enactment but as a way to give my body permission to complete what it could not finish at the time.

By staying present with these sensations in small, manageable doses, I felt the energy move and then settle. My body began to discharge that stored survival energy naturally. This process was quiet, organic, and deeply relieving. Through these sessions, I learned to recognise how my body communicates safety and threat, and how to support myself when activation arises. The gradual restoration of my natural rhythm brought greater confidence, self-trust, and the ability to be present in situations that once felt unbearable.

What I knew in theory, Moniquea helped me put into practice, with tremendous lasting results. I realised that this therapy had helped me become stronger and develop strategies to help me cope with what Brian might say to me at family events.

I'm pleased to say I have been to my first family gathering—a grandchild's birthday party—with Brian and his wife present. Even though I was nervous, I had Ted's support and coped well by not engaging in much conversation with them, but being present and enjoying my family celebration. Another small increment of improvement that is adding up to have an incredibly positive effect.

...woman

...invincible

...strong

...woman

9

MOTHER/DAUGHTER RELATIONSHIP

"If you want to love a parent you have to understand the incredible investment he or she has in you. If you are a parent, and you want to be loved, you have to deserve it."
—Jodi Picoult, *Songs of the Humpback Whale*

THERE WASN'T A DAY that went by during my abusive marriage that I, as a mother, pondered on whether my children were better off without me because I felt so unworthy. It was extremely stressful bringing up my children, all born within four years, who were into everything and required constant attention. The issues with having children close together changed as they grew, but the workload remained incessant.

The pull to get away from the abuse was ever invading my thoughts, but the life calling of responsibility, of remaining to nourish and raise my children was the stronger force. Surviving the birth of the twins had given me the privilege to nurture the lives that had been brought to life from my womb. The bonding I had with each of them from their birth and my love for them was immensely strong. I earnestly felt that they needed their mother. But my doubts of my worthiness and ability to cope in my role as wife and mother was forever in the forefront of my mind. My frequent loss of control and screaming at them to do what I asked was predominately their experience. Proving to my dead grandmother that I wasn't a failure as a wife and a mother pervaded my being, so I stayed. Life went on as ideally as I could make it.

My children became my reason and purpose to stay alive, and through adoring them so much, I continued to live. Giving them life experiences was my agenda: playing sport, learning a musical instrument, play dates with school friends, family holidays, visiting relatives, learning how to cook, youth groups, bike rides together, learning how to tidy and clean their rooms, birthday parties, talking to them about their day at school, problem solving together with issues they were having, the list went on.

Being an involved mother and watching their sport and driving them to their various activities was my life, all the while enduring constant abuse from their father. So why did I stay for so long in an abusive relationship?

Looking back, I've asked myself the same question over and over again. There are many reasons why I stayed as long as I did, and I'm sure there are many reasons why other abused women stay in relationships. Probably the first, and paramount, reason for me was for the children to be with both their parents. I have always felt that children are best nurtured living with both their parents in a loving, encouraging, and supportive environment. When making my wedding vows, I hoped this would be the environment we would create for our family and that I would be married to Brian for the rest of my life. I wanted to honour this vow, even though Brian, by raping me, had broken his vow to me the very day he had made it.

The second reason was financial. In The Age on 11th July 2022, Anne Summers in her article "The choice for many women: violence or poverty," reveals her research into whether there is a bigger problem with "the prevalence of domestic violence in Australia or the consequences for women deciding whether to leave violent relationships." What she found was surprising—that: "It is not poverty that causes domestic violence, as often thought. It is the other way round. Violence causes poverty." I totally agree with her conclusion.

The challenges of being a single parent with teenage children is enough to make any abused woman think twice about embarking on providing for them on her own, albeit with some assistance of child maintenance from their father. I was no different. Brian had been a good provider and I was a stay-at-home mum when the children were small. I had no ability or experience of being able to obtain employment while running the household that matched the income that he was able to bring into the family. This included giving them the most optimum education and various recreational activities that we could afford. By leaving Brian, I would also be leaving the financial support he gave the family, and I was scared I would struggle financially and join the statistics of women in poverty trying to support children on their own.

The third reason I stayed for as long as I did was my on-going hope that he would change, that he would come to his senses and be overwhelmingly sorry for his behaviour and would become the man and husband I believed I had fallen in love with and married. Life would then be happy and exciting, with me being able to cope well and actually be able to enjoy the wonderful children that we had created together. The ramifications of divorce and the effect on the children scared me, plus the shame of being divorced, the feelings of failure, the loss of friends, and the backlash from his family; they all played into my staying.

But after nearly eighteen years of marriage, my hope that Brian would ever change his behaviour towards me—and my optimism that I would be safe if I stayed—began to fade. On top of this, seeing Nathan be physically hurt by his father and finding my mind turning to the terrifying thought of Brian suffocating me with my pillow as I slept, I realised my only choice was to separate. Staying was becoming far too dangerous for all of us and the reasons to stay were overwhelmingly being replaced by my need to be safe and stay alive, especially for the sake of my children.

In her novel *Songs of a Humpback Whale*, Jodi Picoult poignantly explores how unhealed childhood abuse can shape the way a woman mothers her own children. Jane, the main character, endured abuse from her father and later experienced emotional and physical violence in her marriage. At the age of three, her daughter, Rebecca, experienced a horrific accident where she was the only survivor. This incident had kept the family together until, over ten years later, Jane could not stand the treatment any longer and escaped from her husband. But she was unable to escape from her own tormented self. Like so many abused women, she had stayed silent.

The story continues with the three family members dealing with the fallout of their past life experiences, the reasons for their learnt behaviour and the decisions they had made for their lives. It wasn't until another incident occurred where Jane was endeavouring to protect her daughter, that Rebecca reacted, blaming her mother for this incident. Rebecca wanted nothing of her mother. Jane realises that her long held belief that her daughter would just love her unconditionally, simply due to the fact that she was her mother and had given birth to her, was unfounded and that she, as Rebecca's mother, had to earn Rebecca's love and respect. It was at this point that Jane chose to speak and break her silence. In opening up to her daughter, Jane hoped to be understood, and ultimately to be loved, for being a mother *and* for being a woman who had made sacrifices and made choices that she thought was best at the time.

One quote in particular from the novel resonated deeply with me. On page 331, Picoult writes:

> If you want to love a parent you have to understand the incredible investment he or she has in you. If you are a parent, and you want to be loved, you have to deserve it.

The daughter, lying in a hospital bed, couldn't help but listen as her mother told the saga about her own childhood experiences of her father abusing her, and the feelings she had buried along with the abuse of Rebecca's father. She realises her mother had stayed as she was only considering the welfare of her daughter and not her own. Rebecca sympathises and relates to the sacrifice her mother had invested in her and now understands better the reasons for her mother's erratic behaviour, and her own need to be loved and to feel worthy.

Jane concludes that she needs to find a strategy to forgive her father for his abuse and work through her feelings of shame and unworthiness that such abuse had caused, and to resolve to attempt to love herself from now on. The bond between mother and daughter is re-established and strengthened with candour and maturity, arising out of the tragic incident that produced mutual respect.

Picoult writes her mother/daughter storyline using the steps I had realised were necessary for healing lives and relationships. Jane admitted to the abuse by her father that she had locked away, thinking it had no lasting effect on her. But she realised that, even though she had suppressed the memories, the effect on her was still evident. That's why she broke the silence by sharing her story with Rebecca who, ultimately, could then understand the connection with her mother's childhood abuse by her father and how it was influencing her erratic behaviour as a wife and mother. It dawned on Jane that her feelings of imperfection were really feelings of shame that were caused by her father's abuse. It was his guilt, which meant that she could figuratively hand her feelings of shame back to him as his guilt and, at long last, be able to forgive him. Rebecca also followed the steps by admitting to the hurt caused by her mother when she had tried to control Rebecca's choices. Then she also broke the silence of her feelings towards her mother. So, with Jane admitting and apologising to Rebecca for her guilt in the saga and asking Rebecca for forgiveness, which she thankfully gave her mother, the mother/daughter relationship moved toward reconciliation.

Picoult's novel resonated within my soul. The similarity of the mother/daughter bond was palpable with my own. I had expected that Merryn, the precious daughter I had longed for, would love me unconditionally. I was her mother. I gave birth to her and looked after her. Shouting and screaming at my family had become, for me, a necessity that I thought was part of what they had to put up with as one of the struggles of life, just as I had as a child. Brian's passive-aggressive behaviour, of silent response to my attempted communication with him, only antagonised my already frustrated feelings.

At the time, I thought that if they all just did what they were asked to do, I would not need to get upset with them. Connecting the dots between the abuse I suffered at the hands of my grandmother and the deep feelings of low self-esteem and unworthiness it triggered, I came to see how this conditioned me to tolerate Brian's repeated abuse and go into a fawn state—which added to my sense of failure as a wife and mother. This, in turn, only amplified my own behaviour of screaming and yelling when struggling to cope, as I was copying the learnt behaviour of my own mother when she did not cope. This I know caused pain and anxiety to my children, especially Merryn, but I didn't know how to change it as it was so ingrained in my learnt behaviour. Divorce, I believed, caused lifelong issues for children, so I endured the abuse and held on to the hope that it would stop one day.

Like Jane, I did not love myself or feel worthy as a person, largely because of the abuse I endured from my grandmother, the insecurity from my mother's depression, the abuse from my husband, and my belief that I had failed to satisfy my husband and make him happy; they all culminated in a recipe for tragedy. In spite of what I thought of myself at that time, I know I made the right decision to finally leave and remove my children from what I feared would result in disaster.

There are as many sides to every story as there are the individuals concerned. In many cases, there are two people directly involved in the story and then the others affected around the periphery. Everyone is going to have a different interpretation and opinion of events from their own perspective and involvement. Without having the full facts of events, and actually being present at all the experiences, people on the periphery are not going to be able to fully relate to or understand each party's involvement. Making assumptions as to how something happened, or who did what to whom, can distort the actual facts into a totally different scenario.

My children were in the house all the time the abuse was taking place, but they were not in the bedroom with me, and I always tried to be incredibly quiet when the abuse was happening when I was awake. During the day, the frustration I showed progressively toward Brian to try and communicate with him was exasperated by his passive-aggressive silence, which added to my already frustrated state and further inflamed an already tense household. All the children were affected, but especially Merryn, the only girl, who witnessed my continual outbursts of frustration. She surmised that her father, when he was passive and not responding to me, was gentle and unaggressive, which was not the case.

I put my heart and soul into my children. They were my everything and my purpose in life. As their mother, I so wanted to be loved, but I came to believe that the unlovable do not deserve it. Picoult's character, Rebecca, was still living with her mother as a teenager when Jane broke her silence to try to win love and understanding from her daughter. My children are more than double that age. The only way I know to regain trust and love from them has been to start with healing myself. This means speaking out, breaking my silence, admitting and declaring I have been a victim of abuse and naming it as it deserves, and giving back the feelings of shame as the abuser's guilt—as only then can forgiveness work. Then in examining my own conduct, I should also admit to my own errant behaviour that has caused hurt to Brian and the children, apologise to them, ask them for forgiveness, and then change my actions to make it right. This is what I believe is needed to be able to create the possibility for renewal.

So, taking responsibility to break the impasse between us, I wrote Merryn an apology letter, admitting to the hurt I had caused her, apologising for my behaviour, and hoping that she could accept my apology. It was some weeks before her husband, Phil, rang me one evening before handing the phone over to Merryn. We then had a deeply emotional conversation where she verbalised her frustration with me but did say she accepted my apology and forgave me. We have been able to gradually improve our relationship, but I know I will need to put in much more positive action to help rebuild her love and trust in me.

As for my part as a parent with my newfound mantra:

*"If you are a parent and you want to be loved,
you have to deserve it."*

I now desperately want to take responsibility for my part of the relationship and do everything I can possibly do to improve my connection with my children, especially my daughter. As for the other part,

*"If you want to love a parent, you have to understand the
incredible investment he or she has in you."*

I hope that all my children will some day grasp the enormity of the sacrifice I willingly gave of my life to educate them, and to give them fun holidays, sporting and musical experiences, time to talk through their issues and find solutions, help with their homework, and keep them safe in a home that was rife with their father's ongoing abuse of their mother.

I know now that I should have left Brian before they were born, but I didn't, and once they were born, I stayed because of them. I hope that as my children experience their own children growing up, they will realise the huge effort that is required in being a parent, especially as a mother, and the overwhelming sacrifices that you make to give a fulfilling life to your children.

What resonates with me regarding my own scenario of a dysfunctional family that has fallen apart, is the question: *What role, if any, can or should the adult children of a dysfunctional, broken family play in the resolution to a harmonious existence and restoration for everyone?*

This, of course, must be at an appropriate age, and small children should never be used for payback or as weapons of control. Older children, though, can help by using common sense when it comes to disputes but, again, they should never be expected or manipulated into taking sides or being the peacemakers. But if they put their heads in the sand and try to ignore what is going on around them, nobody can gain from an attempt for a successful resolution.

What I asked many times from my young adult children was for them to help me to challenge their father in his behaviour toward me, and be part of making him accountable for his actions. They were never agreeable to this, stating that it was none of their business and up to us as their parents to work out our differences ourselves. I feel strongly that it is also, in part, their business and responsibility. Ultimately, they will benefit from their father being challenged in his behaviour toward their mother if he changes his actions to those of respect and dignity. This would then result in better family functions, where everyone benefits from a harmonious atmosphere where we can enjoy our increasing number of grandchildren (currently nine) together. Not helping me to challenge their father to try and get a positive outcome resulted in me making a statement to the police—a huge step I feel I had to take to try and get some action. But the leopard has not changed his spots, so everyone continues to miss out due to his stubbornness and, maybe, the failure of the legal system to bring him to trial.

Rebecca's father, angry with them both for deserting him, decides to seek them out to bring them back home, but in doing so, he comes to his senses. He admits to himself his selfish and abusive behaviour, acknowledges he needs to be accountable for his actions, and realises his guilt.

Authors of fiction can write a desired outcome for their characters. Real-life sagas, however, have to be played out and experienced with desired results most of the time seemingly unobtainable. Although, I never lose hope that progress can be made and that, one day, a sincere reconciliation between myself and Brian might occur. Such a reconciliation would be so positive for all the expanding family.

...strong
...invincible
...woman

10

ON THE EDGE OF SOMETHING

We're on the edge of something
But we gotta jump now
'Cause we're doing it for them
We're on the edge of something
Possibly beautiful
Possibly beautiful.
—*Edge of Something*, Sung by Missy Higgins
Songwriters: Missy Higgins, Matteo Zingales,
Antony Michael Partos

BACK IN THE 1970S, Helen Reddy's inspiring song *I Am Woman* captured our imagination for hope of a new era, where women could live in a society that would expect gender equality. Motivating words have power when read but when these same words are sung beautifully to inspiring music, the impact can create greater influence and persuasion. Helen Reddy's song has done this. Melodious music along with the message in the words of a song evokes emotions, thoughts, memories, and the felt sense in our bodies. In recent times, Missy Higgins' song *Edge of Something* has also done this, especially for me. It epitomises the energy within me of my resolve for constructive change in society in behaviour towards women and for them to achieve healing, recovery, and accountability.

> *I'm on the edge of something*
> *Got an itch in my bones*
> *There's a fire in the middle of my soul*
> *I'm on the edge of something*
> *And it's gonna take time*
> *But I'm doing it for you*

We must thank all the brave women who courageously came forward with their claims of rape and sexual assault against former Hollywood producer Harvey Weinstein. This eventually resulted in a New York court conviction and a twenty-three-year prison sentence. This fuelled the *#MeToo* movement that had already been started by Tarana Burke. Women came forward with story after story, storming onto the airways exposing controlling and coercive men who denied, denied, denied. This has aided the exposure of the damage done by the "patriarchal society" in all its forms all over the world, and revealed the vast disparity between the genders. Males have manifested disdainful competitiveness against the opposite sex instead of enjoying the innate complementarity of the sexes. Society ought to be more co-operative and recognise the differences between people as a positive. We would all gain the benefit that comes from the various talents and abilities of the complementary gender qualities.

Rather than standing by and witnessing the ongoing power struggle of male strength and control over what the male perceives as the weaker female, I want to be part of changing history for the empowerment of women to be safe in the workplace, on the streets, and in the home. I'm fired up and driven by my own story—my trek—to make a difference by breaking my silence and using my voice for change. Any change to become the expected norm by a progressive society does, however, take time to shift behaviour. But with education and pressure, we can transform expectations for all women now and for future generations of the female gender.

No, no regrets
Got no further to fall
When you've hit the bottom
No, no regrets
I'm my mother's daughter
I got plenty of fight left

I had made a home for Brian and the children, except I was not truly present; only the shell of my body was there. My authentic self—the person I had the potential to be—was not in residence. My mask was on every time I went out of the house; that mask stated that my life was okay as a wife and a mother and that I had everything under control. Yet at home, when the mask was removed, the destructive evidence of who I had become played out in my behaviour within my family. I have no regrets in finally leaving my abusive marriage with my children, as I had no further to fall. Being suicidal, while also fearing being smothered by a pillow at night, was not the way to live a contented life. Either outcome would have been a disaster for everyone in the family, especially for me.

We all are the product of our parents. The influences they have on our upbringing are going to impact our wellbeing for good or bad. It was liberating and life-changing to utilise the "felt sense" to aid in the unpacking of memories and the consequences of having an abusive grandmother and a depressed mother. My mother was affected by her own childhood issues and also suffered from undiagnosed postnatal depression for fifteen years. I am my mother's daughter, and proud to be her daughter, and I have no regrets in having sent my parents a letter describing the effect of her abuse on my child-soul.

I was breaking the silence and enabling conversation and openness in our relationship. That was so healing for the three of us, especially for my mother and myself. Just like Picoult's character Rebecca, who eventually understands the sacrifices made by her mother, I understand the loving sacrifices my own mother made of her time to care for me, teach me life skills, educate me, protect me, and give me memorable childhood experiences, even though she was suffering greatly herself. I am incredibly grateful that she was my mother. I have plenty of fight left in me to help other women break their silence of traumatic childhoods with regard to their mothers and/or grandmothers. I want to use my energy to be part of the restoration of their relationships with the female line of their family, still alive or those who have passed on, so that healing can begin and progress for troubled souls.

I'm on the edge of the unknown
There's a valley of secrets
Stretched out below
But I got you in my chest
And it's giving me power
Yeah, this kinda love don't rest.

Countless women have so many secrets of trauma and abuse that need to be revealed. They need to have the courage, strength, and support to break their silence, so their healing can commence and their fractured relationships can be restored. I stand on the edge of the unknown, uncertain of just how much my strategies for healing will help those who suffer. Even so, I feel empowered to make a difference and show love and support for my fellow-suffering women in whatever way I can.

I wish for perpetrators to be made aware of the damage they have done to the women in their lives, women who should have been able to trust these men. Perpetrators need to admit to their abusive behaviour and apologise, then ask for forgiveness and change their behaviour and actions toward their victims and show them respect and kindness. These men also can be healed from their own guilt and should be encouraging other perpetrators to also reform and be healed.

My resolve is for souls to be on the journey of healing and become stronger, both emotionally and physically, and thus achieve more fulfilling lives and relationships. If only we could all live in a world that is loving and caring toward each other, no matter the gender, rather than competing for superiority, one over the other. The continual persuasion of society, however, still has a long way to go, so we need to keep campaigning for positive change.

No, no regrets
Ain't no further to fall
When you've hit the bottom
No, no regrets
I'm a mother with a daughter
I got plenty of fight left.

Abused women are often too scared to leave an abusive relationship. They fear the reprisal to be worse than the abuse they have been enduring, and are anxious about how they will support and house their children. In recent years, society has started to provide shelters for women and children fleeing abuse, but there is still so much more to be done to provide for the most vulnerable in our communities. I had my family's financial and physical support to be able to set up a new home for my children and myself, but so many who need support don't have family, and even if they do, they are sometimes too proud to ask for help or the family are unable to help. In many cases, abused women are too traumatised to know how to obtain any assistance. Children get caught up in family dysfunction, without any satisfactory solutions available, and can experience more confusion and end up distrusting their parents. Upsetting as this is, it is usually the mother—normally seen by the children to be the nurturer—who becomes the scapegoat, even though she is the one who takes on the care of the children after their parents have split. She can be undermined by a father bent on revenge, which is often unnoticed by the children, who the mother is trying to protect. They listen to a father who either lies or doesn't tell them the full story; he tells them only what he wants them to hear. So, to these children of a broken relationship who are torn between the two disputing parents, the father can seem to be the victim.

Just like Picoult's Jane and Rebecca, there are no easy answers for restoration of the mother/daughter relationship. Yet as its impact goes far beyond the immediate family, it becomes immensely important for a healthy society. I'm a mother with a daughter who I know I have hurt and upset. I also know that I love her more than anything else in this world and I would do anything for her so she may fully comprehend what she means to me. I still hope, fervently, that the prayer I prayed when she was born—that when she was an adult, we would be great friends and share so much of being women together—will come to pass. Even though that prayer has been realised to some extent, my journey to achieve healing and a balanced wellbeing of my mental health has been confusing and bewildering to her. I made a statement to the police about the abuse I received from her father during most of the years of our marriage, but making this statement was not acceptable to her. However I have no regrets. It was time to make a stand and change the lie that I had been telling myself—that I was not worthy of justice. Just as the character Rebecca realises the sacrifices her mother made by returning to her father after the plane crash, my hope is that one day my daughter will realise the sacrifices that I have made. I chose to suffer the enduring, on-going abuse and forfeit the abuse-free life I could have enjoyed if I had left early in the marriage. But I stayed so she and her brothers would be able to have an intact family life with all the benefits that it brought them.

But by staying for as long as I did, the ongoing abuse caused my demeanour to change. I became someone who I would not have naturally been. My behaviour branded me as a deplorable mother, which is such a mistaken and sad outcome. But I did stay, finally leaving once so much damage had been done to me, and the children.

This resulted in a fractured family, with children who, as they got older, did not want to know or understand what caused the fracture. Adult children, I do believe, can have a role to play in obtaining justice and accountability for their abused mothers by challenging their father's denial of responsibility for his behaviour. They need to name abuse to their mothers for what it really is—ABUSE—instead of turning away as if it is none of their business. By saying they don't wish to take sides, they are literally taking the side of the abuser and endorsing the abuse with no accountability. By their lack of involvement, adult children are not only influencing what could be a much more harmonious relationship with their own hostile parents, they are also affecting the plight of other abused women of the next generation. Societal change can come about if adult children make a stand and play their role in bringing about accountability. If they played this positive role, these women—especially mothers with young children—could be saved from violent physical abuse that can go so far as suicide or murder at the hands of their partners. In extreme cases, this can also involve the death of children.

Sexual abuse within families can so easily be hidden from view of the outside world, and yet it is so insidious. Abuse is abuse and it does not matter who has caused that abuse, even if the perpetrator was your father and the victim is your mother. I have plenty of fight left in me to help change our existing culture. Especially now that my mental health has improved, my perspective is that effective and real justice for abused women, particularly abused mothers, is lacking from our legal system. Achieving some sort of justice would then assist in transforming the lives of abused women to some semblance of normality.

So, in answer to my daughter's statements and questions to me from Chapter 2: *Mum! What do you think you are doing? What about forgiveness? What good will come of going to the police? He's my dad!* My aims have many aspects.

So, my answer is as follows:

First, I wanted to start the process of healing from my PTSD as remaining silent hadn't worked for me. I wanted to be heard and believed about the abuse I had endured. I wanted my statement to become part of the statistics that show the extent of the problem our society is enduring of sexual abuse towards women from intimate partners. All these aims I have achieved.

Second, forgiveness wasn't enough to achieve relief from the abuse I had endured, and I needed to discover more ways to find answers for healing. By going to the police, I forged a new path of revelation and energy that enabled me to find additional answers so I could attain a successful solution to commence my recovery process. To only rely on forgiveness to achieve positive results wasn't enough for me. This aim I have achieved.

And third, so much good has come from going to the police. My awareness of the injustice against women has expanded. I now want to assist with constructive change in our society. I started to write down my thoughts, which eventually expanded into this book. Writing down my thoughts made me go looking for information to better understand how we, as human beings, can instinctively function when confronted with trauma, and how we can use this understanding to be able to forge a path towards recovery. I have successfully transformed myself into a "sexual abuse overcomer."

Brian is now on the Sex Offender's Register. Even though he wasn't taken to trial due to insufficient evidence to achieve a conviction beyond reasonable doubt, the detectives said that as I had made a substantial complaint, he was automatically put on that watch list. So this aim was partially successful.

What I didn't achieve, though, was to make Brian accountable for his treatment of me. All I wanted was a wholehearted admission of guilt, a genuine apology, and for him to ask to be forgiven and start treating me with the respect, honour, and dignity that the mother of his children deserves. I would also like him to confess to the children what he really did to me, apologise, ask for their forgiveness, and change his behaviour so we can all enjoy our children and grandchildren together.

Just because he is their father does not exempt him from being accountable for his actions toward their mother—abuse is abuse and needs to be called out for what it is: ABUSE! By going to the police, women push for justice and accountability. But justice is very hard to achieve within our legal system as cases generally end up as a "he said/she said" case, resulting in the prosecuting authority believing that there is insufficient evidence for them to go to trial. This is what happened in my case.

A victim should be given protection through our legal system so they can feel safe in the community. If a perpetrator is found guilty by the court, a decent prison sentence needs to be given to serve as a deterrent for other potential perpetrators. However, accountability has more personal benefit for a victim. If a perpetrator has any conscience, when questioned by the police he should see the destructiveness of his exploits, plead guilty, suffer the consequences, and change his behaviour towards his victim. This would be the desired result for a better life for everyone involved. Also, when pleading guilty and receiving a more favourable victim impact statement, a court would be more likely to impose a lighter sentence.

So, I partially achieved my desired outcome by making a statement to the police. I feel substantially positive that it was the right action and so I am pleased that I decided to do it. I am achieving a better balanced and contented life.

My hope, however, is to still achieve harmony within my family for the sake of the children, grandchildren, and for the sake of Deirdre and Brian.

Hope is a powerful feeling.

Everybody gonna know my name
I'll be the one with the heart on fire
Screaming from the highest stage
Everybody gonna know my name
'Cause I'm the girl who's gonna be everything
that's ever made you afraid
Hell hath no fury like a woman's rage
Everybody gonna know my name
Everybody gonna know my name
Everybody gonna know my name
Everybody gonna know my name
Everybody gonna know my...

In her speech, when accepting the Cecil B. De Mille Award at the Golden Globes in 2018, Oprah Winfrey said:

"So, I want tonight to express gratitude to all the women who have endured years of abuse and assault because they, like my mother, had children to feed and bills to pay and dreams to pursue. They're the women whose names we will never know."

There are so many names we will never know of women who suffered in silence, who were trying to feed their children, pay the bills, and pursue their dreams whilst enduring abuse. Sadly, most have ended up having no voice at all. Some who have died at the hands of their perpetrators may make it into the news, but most slip by without any acknowledgement or recognition.

Just as Oprah was proud of the women who had come forward with their stories, I too am grateful for those women in Australia whose names we do know, who have felt strong enough and empowered enough to come forward. These are the women who have spoken up about their experiences. These are the women who have a strong desire for change and justice, even in some cases putting their careers on the line.

Let's make the male gender of our species afraid as we unleash the fire in our hearts, with a collective rage of women through the media, of our anger at the treatment of women and their children. Abused women all have names, and all have stories to tell. Let's break the silence so men will fathom the potential damage they are causing to their families and to society in general. It's time for constructive change, justice, and accountability.

We're on the edge of something
But we gotta jump now
'Cause we're doing it for them
We're on the edge of something
Possibly beautiful
Possibly beautiful

Society as a whole is on the "edge of something," but we do need to make huge changes if we are going to prevent more women being badly affected by abuse or even losing their lives. We need to do it now. Young girls and boys growing up need to be educated about how to expect to be treated and how to behave around the opposite sex. Homes and schools need to take action and be proactive in promoting societal change and expectations. The media needs to stop using the word "survivor" when it comes to speaking about sexual abuse as it is fuelling the wrong message about victims. This wrong usage is hampering victims' recovery. Once a victim has taken ownership of the fact that they have been a victim and worked through all its implications, to be called a "survivor" anchors them in the "victim stage." Instead, they should be called "sexual abuse endurers" who will then, hopefully, move along the journey of healing and become "sexual abuse overcomers."

As Osborne-Crowley says, there will not be a time that she is not "recovering" from her experience of sexual abuse. So, in my language, she is continually "overcoming."

I have been a Sexual Abuse Endurer, but now I am a Sexual Abuse Overcomer. There will never be a time that I'm not overcoming this abuse, but I have learnt how to manage my PTSD and I am now content with life. I want other women to become Sexual Abuse Overcomers too. We need to hold on to the hope of being overcomers, as this realisation could make life "possibly beautiful."

...invincible

...strong

...woman

REFERENCES

American Psychiatric Association. 2022. *Diagnostic and Statistical Manual of Mental Disorders*. 5th ed., Text Revision. Arlington, VA: American Psychiatric Publishing.

ANROWS (Australia's National Research Organisation for Women's Safety).

Australian Domestic and Family Violence Death Review Network, and Australia's National Research Organisation for Women's Safety. *Australian Domestic and Family Violence Death Review Network Data Report: Intimate Partner Violence Homicides 2010–2018*. 2nd ed.; Research Report 03/2022. Sydney: ANROWS, 2022.

Arndt, Bettina, 'Nicolass Bester and Bettina Arndt Interview, FEMINIST CENSORSHIP Grace Tame' *Youtube*.

Coughlin, Deborah, *Outspoken: 50 Speeches By Incredible Women*. London: WH Allen, 2019.

Ferrante, Elena, *My Brilliant Friend*. English Translation, Ann Goldstein. Melbourne, Victoria: The Text Publishing Company, 2016.

Ferrante, Elena, *The Story of A New Name*. English Translation, Ann Goldstein. Melbourne, Victoria: The Text Publishing Company, 2019.

Ferrante, Elena, *Those Who Leave And Those Who Stay*. English Translation, Ann Goldstein. Melbourne, Victoria: The Text Publishing Company, 2019.

Ferrante, Elena, *The Story Of The Lost Child*. English Translation, Ann Goldstein. Melbourne, Victoria: The Text Publishing Company, 2019.

Higgins, Melissa and Zingales, Matteo and Partos, Antony Michael. 'Missy Higgins - Edge of Something' *Musixmatch*. Edge of Something lyrics [©] Hipgnosis Beats.

Kantor, Jodi and Twohey, Megan, *She Said: Breaking The Sexual Harassment Story That Helped Ignite A Movement.* London: Bloomsbury Circus, 2019.

Kroeger, Catherine Clark and Nason-Clark, Nancy, *No Place For Abuse: Biblical and Practical Resources to Counteract Domestic Violence.* Downers Grove, Illinois: InterVarsity Press, 2010.

Lee, Nicole, 'Nicole Lee – Disability Advocacy Resource Unit (DARU)'.

Levine, Peter A., *Waking the Tiger: Healing Trauma.* Berkeley, California: North Atlantic Books, 1997.

Milligan, Louise, 'Inside the Canberra Bubble' *Four Corners - ABC.* 9 Nov 2020,.

Milligan, Louise, 'I am That Girl' *Four Corners – ABC.* 7 May 2018.

Moriarty, Liane, *Big Little Lies.* Sydney, New South Wales: Pan Macmillan Australia, 2018.

Mullins, Saxon, 'Rape & Sexual Assault Research & Advocacy' Feb 2020.

Osborne-Crowley, Lucia, *I Choose Elena.* Crows Nest, New South Wales: Allen & Unwin, 2020.

Osborne-Crowley, Lucia, *My Body Keeps Your Secrets.* Crows Nest, New South Wales: Allen & Unwin, 2021.

Picoult, Jodi, *Songs of The Humpback Whale.* Crows Nest, New South Wales: Allen & Unwin, 2003.

Reddy, Helen and Burton, Ray, 'Helen Reddy – I Am Woman (1971)' *Musixmatch.* I am Woman lyrics © Buggerlugs Music Co., Irving Music, Inc. https://www.youtube.com/watch?v=ZrVLL7soS1U

Resick, Patricia A., Monson, Candice M. and Chard, Kathleen M., *Cognitive Processing Therapy for PTSD, A Comprehensive Manual.* New York, NY: The Guilford Press, 2017.

Rothschild, Babette, *The Body Remembers: The Psychophysiology of Trauma and Trauma Treatment.* New York: W. W. Norton & Company, 2000.

Royal Commission into Family Violence. Report and Recommendations. Melbourne: State of Victoria, 2016.

Royal Commission into Institutional Responses to Child Sexual Abuse. *Final Report*. Canberra: Commonwealth of Australia, 2017.

Spiteri, A. Moniquea, 'Somatic Therapy: The Key to Overcoming Trauma'.

Summers, Anne, 'The choice for many women: violence or poverty' The Age, Melbourne, 11 July 2022, p .19.

Tame, Grace, 'Grace Tame Advocate for Survivors of Sexual Assault – Australian of the Year 2021'.

Truu, Maani, 'Disability: Women with disability are being turned away by family violence services in Australia' *SBS News.* 25 Nov 2020,

Whitburn, Michaela, "Insulting': Saxon Mullins takes aim at sexual consent reform plan" *The Sydney Morning Herald*. 21 Nov 2020.

Winfrey, Oprah. *Acceptance Speech at the 75th Golden Globe Awards*. Beverly Hills, CA, January 7, 2018. Accessed February 2025.

Resources

CASA – Centre Against Sexual Assault

Services for crisis support for sexual assault and for access to ongoing counselling.

For Crisis Support Call: 1800 806 292

For Counselling Support Call: 03 9635 3610 (Melbourne, Australia)

www.casahouse.com.au

1800RESPECT

Australia's national domestic, family and sexual violence counselling , information and support service.

Call: 1800 737 732

www.1800respect.org.au

Lifeline

A national charity providing all Australians experiencing emotional distress with access to 24-hour crisis support and suicide prevention services.

Call: 13 11 14

www.lifeline.org.au

Relationships Australia

Supports the nurturing of relationships for both individual mental health and general community outcomes so that everyone can build and maintain respect in their relationships.

Call: 1300 364 277

www.relationships.com.au

Beyond Blue

For mental health support when you may need to talk to someone who can help or connect with others online in a forum anonymously.

Call: 1300 224 636

www.beyondblue.org.au

General contacts that may direct you to your state or local area.

ACKNOWLEDGEMENTS

It seems odd to make an acknowledgement to a virus, but I need to claim that if it hadn't been for the COVID-19 pandemic, this book probably would never have been written. Being locked away at home with the time to immerse myself into research of trauma by sexual abuse enabled me to develop my thinking and put the words together on my computer.

Throughout this time, the main person who constantly encouraged me was Ted, my husband of fifteen years. He would read and comment on what I had written, make suggestions for improvement, and continue to urge me to keep writing. His continual support throughout my diagnosis of PTSD and the on-going treatments has strengthened my desire for life and to live it to the fullest. Without his love and support I wouldn't be who I am today.

I would like to thank my cousin Janine who, being a counsellor, has been an encouraging voice at the end of the phone when I have been at low points in my life. Her solid resolve in being positive with what we can work on and leave alone what we cannot change has been very helpful. Loaning me her many books on trauma inspired me to investigate further into the diagnosis and treatments portrayed by Peter Levine and his theories on somatic therapy. This research made me investigate the treatment for myself and that's when I found Moniquea, my Somatic Psychotherapist.

My gratitude goes to Moniquea in enabling me to put into practice what I had researched about somatic therapy. She taught me the benefit of understanding my body sensations to release the locked away effects of trauma on my life. Not only did she do this but put me in touch with my wonderful editor, Ruth Fae.

Ruth has ordered my words into shape to make my writing resemble what a proper book should be like. Both of us being women who have experienced trauma from a person who should have loved us the most, we have had a kindred spirit and our words sing the same song. For this connection and empathy, I have been most grateful as it has been valuable in our discussions for her to make my trek into being readable.

To my parents, I thank them for their unwavering support and encouragement of me throughout the turbulent years of the collapse of my first marriage and with my children, who they adored. With losing Mum in the last few years, Dad has continued to encourage me to get on with enjoying living life, being positive about my opening up about my struggles, but also my successes, by putting them into written words.

My sister, Jay (Jacqueline), has always been in my life. Growing up, we enjoyed many holidays with our parents, either at the beach where we sailed together, or out in the wide-open countryside of Australia. She has continued to be a great travelling companion as we venture out to experience fascinating destinations, either to sightsee or to challenge ourselves to walking adventures. I value her company on our expeditions that are tremendous for improving my mental health and wellbeing. Thanks also for your efforts with the photography for the front cover.

I'm so proud of my three boys, Nathan, Jared, and Rohan who have turned out to be fine young men, even with the chaotic childhood they experienced. As their mother, who loves them so, so much, I wish to thank them for standing by me, even though at times I wasn't very loveable.

However, the most passionate acknowledgement I want to make is to the most important woman in my life, my precious daughter, Merryn. She has courageously agreed to allow me to use the chapter I wrote from her point of view of her experience of having parents who were fighting and yelling throughout her childhood. I am so grateful for her permission to bare her life so that my trek has the balance that I wanted it to have by adding the details from a child's point of view, especially as the only girl in the family. Her bravery has strengthened our relationship, and I hope will help other families to restore relationships and find healing in their lives too. I love you so much, Merryn.

Author Bio

About Deirdre Fennessy

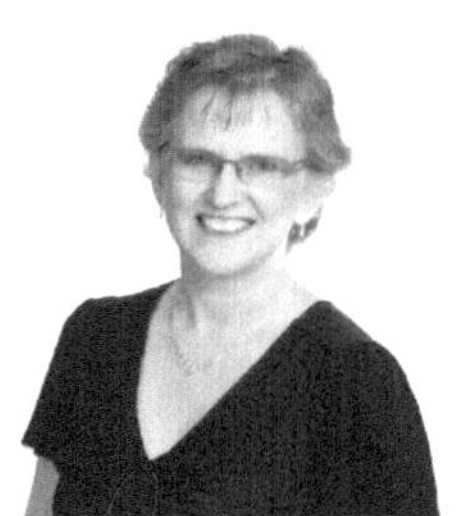

DEIRDRE FENNESSY IS A first-time author whose writing is grounded in truth, resilience, and a deep desire to make a difference through speaking her truth. Her debut memoir, "*Mum, He's My Dad!*" is the result of years spent coming to terms with the abuse she endured in childhood and during her first marriage. By sharing her story, Deirdre hopes to break generational cycles of silence and empower others to recognise their own worth, voice, and capacity for healing.

With a background in pastoral care, Deirdre has spent decades supporting others through life's most vulnerable moments. She believes that listening deeply to people's stories has strengthened her understanding of the uniqueness and dignity of every person's journey. As an Authorised Marriage Celebrant, she brings empathy, insight, and integrity to each ceremony, honouring the relationships and transitions that shape our lives.

Deirdre lives on Victoria's beautiful Mornington Peninsula with her husband, Ted. When she's not writing, she enjoys playing tennis, walking in nature, and travelling across Australia and the world. She treasures time with her four adult children, their partners, and her nine beloved grandchildren—the next generation for whom she writes and hopes.